Health Freedom: Navigating Wellness Autonomy Using Internet Resources, Blood Chemistry Insight, and Secured Surgery, Dentistry Plus Cancer Healthcare Accesses

By Meklit Garedew Gebrewold

© 2024 by Meklit Garedew

Cover design by Meklit Garedew Gebrewold

Meklit Garedew Gebrewold's contact: meklitgara91@gmail.com

Introduction

In today's digital era, individuals are bestowed with unparalleled authority to seize control of their health and well-being. Within the vast expanse of online resources lies the power for people to equip themselves with the knowledge necessary to emerge as the primary architects of their wellness journey. This elevated sense of proactive self-care inaugurates a transformative era in healthcare dynamics, granting individuals the ability to engage in informed dialogues with healthcare professionals, take active roles in pivotal healthcare decisions, and sculpt bespoke health strategies harmonized with their unique needs and preferences.

This enlightening book amplifies the discourse on how individuals can wield this empowerment to autonomously steward their health, reserving the prerogative to direct their well-being until circumstances escalate to a critical juncture necessitating professional intervention. By advocating for self-reliance and embracing proactive health management, the narrative champions the notion of individuals assuming the mantle of their health destiny. This approach nurtures a profound sense of health sovereignty, endowing individuals with the autonomy to make discerning choices concerning their health without sole reliance on external directives.

At the core of this narrative is the profound recognition of utilizing tools such as blood chemistry tests as a strategic mechanism for individuals to embody their health freedom. The book intricately explores how these tests serve as formidable allies in the pursuit of optimal health, rendering invaluable insights into one's physiological status and catalyzing the cultivation of detailed health enhancement blueprints. By accentuating the pivotal role of these tests in empowering individuals to monitor, comprehend, and optimize their health trajectory, the book exalts the transformative potential engendered through embracing self-guided health management. Moreover, the book underscores the crucial importance for governments to fortify the security and efficacy of surgery, dentistry, and cancer healthcare systems, stipulating that legal healthcare facilities should be sought for such specialized services, affirming the paramount significance of safeguarding these critical healthcare domains.

Contents

1. Chapter One: The Power of Self-Advocacy and Internet Empowerment
2. Chapter Two: Empowering Ourselves through Self-Care and Online Resources

3. Chapter Three: Empowering Health Freedom: Navigating Healthcare Challenges and Avoiding Medicine-Based Criminal Activities Through Self-Care and Internet Research
4. Chapter Four: Empowering Self-Care: A Path to Health Freedom and Legal Recognition
5. Chapter Five: Empowering Health Freedom: Liberating Individuals through Knowledge and Autonomy
6. Chapter Six: Empowering Health Literacy: Navigating the Digital Landscape for Accurate Diagnosis and Wellness
7. Chapter Seven: Safeguarding Health: Navigating Risks and Empowering Choices Through Online Resources
8. Chapter Eight: Empowering Health Literacy: Navigating Knowledge in the Digital Age
9. Chapter Nine: Embracing Knowledge for Personal Empowerment
10. Chapter Ten: Empowering Health Autonomy: Navigating Wellness Through Online Resources
11. Chapter Eleven: Guiding Light: Navigating Healthcare Insecurities and Embracing Health Freedom
12. Chapter Twelve: Futuristic Healthcare Horizons: Governments Leading the Way with Advanced Laboratory Services and High-Tech Tools
13. Chapter Thirteen: Vital Insights: The Whispering Truth within Our Veins Revealed through Blood Chemistry
14. Chapter Fourteen: Empowering Health Freedom: Government-Driven Healthcare Security in Surgical, Dental, and Cancer Services

Chapter One: The Power of Self-Advocacy and Internet Empowerment

The remarkable advancement of the internet has transformed the way people access information. In the realm of healthcare, individuals are increasingly empowered to take charge of their well-being by harnessing the wealth of knowledge available online. The internet has become a gateway to a vast repository of medical literature, research studies, and expert opinions, enabling individuals to educate themselves about various health conditions and treatments. This newfound accessibility to information has elevated the concept of self-advocacy, offering individuals the opportunity to proactively manage their health.

In the age of digital empowerment, individuals are no longer just passive recipients of medical advice. Armed with internet resources, people have the potential to become informed and proactive participants in their healthcare journey. By leveraging the internet, individuals can research their symptoms, understand potential diagnoses, and explore treatment options. The ability to conduct thorough research about one's health concerns creates a paradigm shift, allowing individuals to make more informed decisions about their healthcare.

One of the most significant advantages of using the internet as a healthcare resource is the opportunity to adopt self-care strategies. When individuals delve into the depths of online information, they often discover valuable insights into maintaining and improving their health. In the context of becoming one's own doctor, the internet serves as a platform for individuals to explore a wide array of self-care practices, from healthy lifestyle habits to evidence-based holistic remedies. The wealth of self-help materials available on the internet, including e-books, articles, and reputable websites, equips individuals with the knowledge and tools to take charge of their well-being.

Moreover, by utilizing internet resources, individuals can gain a comprehensive understanding of their health conditions, allowing them to engage in more meaningful discussions with healthcare professionals. Armed with knowledge acquired from reputable online sources, individuals can articulate their concerns and questions more effectively during medical appointments. This enhanced communication facilitates a collaborative approach to healthcare, where individuals actively contribute to the decision-making process regarding their treatment plans.

Embracing the role of one's own healthcare advocate through internet-enabled self-education opens the door to a myriad of opportunities for optimizing health outcomes. Harnessing the power of internet resources empowers individuals to adopt proactive measures such as preventive screenings, early intervention, and lifestyle modifications, all of which contribute to the promotion of overall wellness. By becoming active participants in their healthcare journey, individuals can leverage the internet to access evidence-based recommendations and practical strategies for promoting their own well-being.

It is essential to recognize that the internet, with its abundance of information, also necessitates discernment and critical thinking. While the internet offers a wealth of valuable medical knowledge, it is imperative for individuals to navigate this vast landscape with caution and discretion. Engaging with credible sources, verifying information, and seeking professional guidance when necessary are integral aspects of utilizing the internet as a tool for self-care and medical exploration.

The internet serves as a catalyst for democratizing healthcare information, empowering individuals to transcend traditional barriers and take ownership of their health. This newfound capacity to be one's own doctor, to an extent, revolutionizes the dynamics of healthcare, fostering a culture of informed autonomy and proactive self-advocacy.

As we embark on this journey of self-discovery and health empowerment through the internet, it is essential to approach the wealth of available information with a sense of responsibility and empowerment, recognizing the potential to transform our health and well-being through knowledge and informed decision-making.

The internet has emerged as a powerful ally in the quest for self-health management, offering individuals the tools and resources to become active participants in their healthcare journey. By harnessing the wealth of information available online and leveraging self-care strategies through internet resources, individuals are poised to redefine their roles as informed advocates for their own well-being. This chapter lays the foundation for embracing the transformative potential of internet-enabled self-advocacy, setting the stage for a journey of empowerment, knowledge, and proactive health management.

The rapid and pervasive advancement of the internet has revolutionized the landscape of healthcare, offering individuals unprecedented access to a vast reservoir of medical information. Through online platforms, people can now delve into a plethora of medical literature, research findings, and expert insights, empowering them to become proactive agents in managing their health and well-being. This paradigm shift towards internet-enabled self-advocacy marks a significant evolution in healthcare dynamics, emphasizing the pivotal role of informed decision-making and autonomy in one's health journey.

The democratization of knowledge facilitated by the internet has elevated individuals from passive recipients to active participants in healthcare. By leveraging online resources, individuals can delve deep into their symptoms, investigate potential diagnoses, and explore various treatment alternatives. This newfound capacity to educate oneself about health conditions not only fosters a sense of empowerment but also enables individuals to make more informed choices regarding their healthcare, thereby driving a more engaged approach to personal well-being.

One of the key strengths of utilizing the internet as a healthcare tool lies in its ability to promote self-care practices. Through online research, individuals can uncover a treasure trove of information on healthy lifestyle choices, wellness strategies, and evidence-based interventions. By immersing themselves in a plethora of self-help materials available online, ranging from articles to e-books, individuals can equip themselves with the knowledge and insights necessary to proactively manage and enhance their health, bolstering the concept of self-directed healthcare.

Harnessing internet resources enables individuals to deepen their understanding of specific health conditions, thereby facilitating more meaningful and productive dialogues with healthcare professionals. Armed with knowledge gleaned from reputable online sources, individuals can effectively communicate their concerns, share insights, and actively participate in shaping their treatment plans. This collaborative engagement between individuals and healthcare providers, underpinned by informed internet research, paves the way for a more patient-centric and holistic approach to healthcare delivery.

The embrace of self-advocacy through internet-enabled self-education unlocks a myriad of possibilities for optimizing health outcomes and fostering overall wellness. By leveraging online resources, individuals can proactively engage in preventive measures, early interventions, and lifestyle modifications, all of which are integral components of a comprehensive approach to well-being. The internet acts as a gateway to evidence-based recommendations and practical tools that individuals can harness to promote their health and vitality, accentuating the role of proactive self-management in health maintenance.

Nevertheless, amidst the wealth of information available online, it is essential for individuals to exercise discernment and critical thinking. While the internet provides a wealth of valuable medical insights, ensuring the credibility and reliability of sources, as well as seeking professional guidance when needed, are crucial aspects of navigating the digital healthcare landscape responsibly. By cultivating a vigilant approach to online health information, individuals can make informed decisions and mitigate the risks of misinformation or inappropriate self-diagnosis.

The internet serves as a catalyst for democratizing healthcare information, transcending traditional boundaries and empowering individuals to take ownership of their health and well-being. This shift towards internet-enabled self-advocacy not only reshapes the dynamics of healthcare delivery but also nurtures a culture of informed autonomy and proactive engagement with one's health. By embracing the role of one's own healthcare advocate, individuals can leverage the power of the internet to embark on a journey of self-discovery, empowerment, and personalized health management.

The chapter commences by highlighting the transformative impact of the internet on information accessibility, especially within the healthcare landscape. It stresses how the internet has emerged as a pivotal tool in empowering individuals to actively engage in managing their well-being. This empowerment is reinforced by the abundance of medical literature, research studies, and expert opinions available online, which enables individuals to educate themselves about various health conditions and treatments.

The chapter emphasizes that individuals are no longer passive recipients of medical advice but active participants in their healthcare journey. It underscores the significance of the internet in enabling individuals to conduct thorough research about their health concerns, thereby facilitating more informed decisions about their healthcare. By leveraging internet resources, individuals can explore symptoms, potential diagnoses, and treatment options, thereby transforming their role from mere patients to informed decision-makers regarding their health.

The chapter delves into the concept of self-care strategies and how the internet serves as a platform for individuals to access a wide array of self-help materials. It underscores the importance of individuals being able to explore various self-care practices and gain insights into maintaining and improving their health through reputable online sources.

The chapter also discusses the positive impact of internet-enabled self-education on improving communication between individuals and healthcare professionals. It highlights how individuals, armed with knowledge acquired from credible online sources, can articulate their concerns and questions more effectively during medical appointments, leading to a more collaborative approach to healthcare decision-making.

Moreover, the chapter emphasizes the opportunities for optimizing health outcomes that arise from individuals becoming their own healthcare advocates. It underscores how harnessing the power of internet resources empowers individuals to adopt proactive measures, such as preventive screenings, early intervention, and lifestyle modifications, for the promotion of overall wellness.

It also responsibly acknowledges the need for discernment and critical thinking when navigating the wealth of information available on the internet. It stresses the importance of engaging with credible sources, verifying information, and seeking professional guidance when necessary, thus emphasizing the need for caution and discretion while utilizing the internet as a tool for self-care and medical exploration.

The chapter highlights the internet as a catalyst for democratizing healthcare information, empowering individuals to transcend traditional barriers and take ownership of their health. It discusses how this newfound capacity to be one's own doctor revolutionizes the dynamics of healthcare, fostering a culture of informed autonomy and proactive self-advocacy.

This first chapter effectively outlines the transformative impact of the internet on healthcare consumerism, advocating for informed self-advocacy and demonstrating the potential of internet empowerment to facilitate proactive engagement in personal health management. It emphasizes the need for caution, critical thinking, and responsible utilization of online resources while recognizing the opportunities for improving individual health outcomes through active participation in healthcare decisions.

The remarkable advancement of the internet has paved the way for a paradigm shift in how people access information. This holds especially true within the realm of healthcare, where individuals are increasingly empowered to take charge of their well-being by utilizing the vast reservoir of knowledge available online. The internet has become a gateway to a wealth of medical literature, research studies, and expert opinions, allowing individuals to educate themselves about various health conditions and available treatments. This newfound accessibility to information has elevated the concept of self-advocacy, offering individuals the opportunity to actively participate in managing their health proactively.

In the age of digital empowerment, individuals are no longer just passive recipients of medical advice. Armed with internet resources, people have the potential to become informed and proactive participants in their healthcare journey. By leveraging the internet, individuals can research their symptoms, understand potential diagnoses, and explore treatment options. The ability to conduct thorough research about one's health concerns creates a paradigm shift, allowing individuals to make more informed decisions about their healthcare.

One of the most significant advantages of utilizing the internet as a healthcare resource is the opportunity to adopt self-care strategies. When individuals delve into the depths of online information, they often discover valuable insights into maintaining and improving their health. In the context of becoming one's own doctor, the internet serves as a platform for individuals to explore a wide array of self-care practices, from healthy lifestyle habits to evidence-based holistic remedies. The wealth of self-help materials available on the internet, including e-books, articles, and reputable websites, equips individuals with the knowledge and tools to take charge of their well-being.

Moreover, by utilizing internet resources, individuals can gain a comprehensive understanding of their health conditions, allowing them to engage in more meaningful discussions with healthcare professionals. Armed with knowledge acquired from reputable online sources, individuals can articulate their concerns and questions more effectively during medical appointments. This enhanced communication facilitates a collaborative approach to healthcare, where individuals actively contribute to the decision-making process regarding their treatment plans.

Embracing the role of one's own healthcare advocate through internet-enabled self-education opens the door to a myriad of opportunities for optimizing health outcomes. Harnessing the power of internet resources empowers individuals to adopt proactive measures such as preventive screenings, early intervention, and lifestyle modifications, all of which contribute to the promotion of overall wellness. By becoming active participants in their healthcare journey, individuals can leverage the internet to access evidence-based recommendations and practical strategies for promoting their own well-being.

It is essential to recognize that the internet, with its abundance of information, also necessitates discernment and critical thinking. While the internet offers a wealth of valuable medical knowledge, it is imperative for individuals to navigate this vast landscape with caution and discretion. Engaging with credible sources, verifying information, and seeking professional guidance when necessary are integral aspects of utilizing the internet as a tool for self-care and medical exploration.

The internet serves as a catalyst for democratizing healthcare information, empowering individuals to transcend traditional barriers and take ownership of their health. This newfound capacity to be one's own doctor, to an extent, revolutionizes the dynamics of healthcare, fostering a culture of informed autonomy and proactive self-advocacy.

Chapter Two: Empowering Ourselves through Self-Care and Online Resources

In today's fast-paced world, where immediate access to information is at our fingertips, the power of self-care and self-empowerment has never been more achievable. Waiting for specialized medical professionals to provide care can often lead to delays in treatment and unnecessary stress. By taking charge of our health and well-being, we can effectively utilize our time and resources to address our health concerns promptly and proactively.

The internet, a vast repository of knowledge and information, serves as a valuable tool in empowering individuals to take control of their health. With just a simple search, one can gain access to a wealth of information on various health conditions, symptoms, treatments, and preventive measures. By educating ourselves about our health through reliable online sources, we can make informed decisions that positively impact our well-being.

Engaging in self-research about illnesses and medical conditions empowers individuals to become their own health advocates. By leveraging the plethora of resources available online, such as reputable medical websites, forums, and e-books, individuals can equip themselves with the knowledge needed to understand their symptoms, explore treatment options, and make informed decisions about their health.

Utilizing the internet to research health-related topics allows individuals to develop personalized strategies for managing their health effectively. By accessing e-books and online resources that offer insights into holistic approaches to wellness, individuals can tailor their self-care routines to meet their specific needs and preferences. This personalized approach can lead to improved health outcomes and a greater sense of empowerment over one's well-being.

Moreover, by becoming knowledgeable about their health and utilizing online resources effectively, individuals can also contribute to building a healthier society. Empowered individuals who take active roles in their health not only benefit themselves but also create pressure for healthcare systems and governments to provide accessible and effective healthcare services. This shift towards self-care and self-advocacy can lead to the development of simplified and safer healthcare pathways that prioritize individual well-being and health freedom.

Governments can harness the power of online resources and self-care initiatives to promote public health awareness and education. By encouraging individuals to take an active role in their health and providing support for online health resources, governments can empower citizens to make informed decisions about their well-being. This collaborative approach can lead to the development of user-friendly healthcare solutions that cater to the diverse needs of the population, fostering a culture of health and self-responsibility.

By embracing the concept of being our own doctors through internet research and self-education, individuals can take proactive steps towards maintaining their health and well-being. Through a combination of self-care practices, online resources, and informed decision-making, individuals can navigate the complexities of healthcare systems with confidence and autonomy. This shift towards self-empowerment in healthcare not only benefits individuals on a personal level but also contributes to the greater goal of creating a society where health freedom and well-being are paramount.

The utilization of online resources and self-care practices can empower individuals to take control of their health and lead fulfilling lives. By leveraging the wealth of information available on the internet, individuals can become their own health advocates, make informed decisions about their well-being, and contribute to a healthier society. Governments can support this paradigm shift by promoting public health awareness and providing accessible healthcare solutions that prioritize individual empowerment and health freedom. Empowering ourselves through self-care and online resources is not just a trend but a transformative approach towards living a life of holistic health and well-being.

Empowering ourselves to take control of our health and well-being is a remarkable step towards self-care and self-sufficiency. In today's digital age, the internet serves as a vast reservoir of knowledge and resources that we can utilize to better understand our health needs. Waiting for specialized medical professionals can sometimes be time-consuming and overwhelming, but by taking initiative and utilizing the plethora of information available online, we can expedite our healthcare journey.

When we intricately research our symptoms or potential illnesses on the internet, we are equipping ourselves with the tools necessary to make informed decisions regarding our health. Various reputable websites, medical journals, and forums provide valuable information that can assist us in understanding our conditions better. By utilizing these online resources, we can bridge the gap between seeking professional medical help and taking control of our health independently.

The accessibility of e-books and online publications allows us to delve deeper into specific conditions, treatments, and preventive measures. By educating ourselves through these resources, we can equip ourselves with the knowledge needed to make sound choices for our health. This self-learning approach not only saves time but also promotes a sense of self-reliance and empowerment in managing our well-being.

By being proactive in our health management through online research and education, we are essentially becoming our own doctors in a digital sense. Harnessing the power of the internet enables us to adopt best practices and strategies tailored to our individual health needs. This personalized approach not only enhances our understanding of medical conditions but also helps us make well-informed decisions regarding our health.

The utilization of internet resources for health-related information can have broader implications at a societal level. By promoting self-care and self-empowerment through digital platforms, governments can encourage their citizens to take charge of their health outcomes. By emphasizing the importance and reliability of online health resources, governments can cultivate a culture of health consciousness and autonomy within their populations.

Creating simple and safe pathways for individuals to access accurate health information online can revolutionize the way people perceive and interact with healthcare. By facilitating user-friendly platforms and promoting trustworthy sources, governments can empower individuals to lead healthier lives independently. This shift not only reduces the burden on healthcare systems but also fosters a sense of responsibility and ownership over personal health.

In essence, by embracing the role of our own health advocates and leveraging the internet as a powerful tool, we can proactively manage our well-being more effectively. From researching symptoms to exploring treatment options and preventive strategies, the digital landscape offers a wealth of information that can guide us towards better health outcomes. By embracing self-care and utilizing online resources wisely, we not only benefit individually but also contribute to a more informed and health-conscious society.

Utilizing the resources available on the internet for health-related information and self-care can empower individuals to take charge of their own health and well-being, leading to more effective use of time and a proactive approach to self-care. By accessing online resources, individuals can gain knowledge about various health conditions and treatments without having to wait for an appointment with a specialized healthcare provider. This can enable them to make informed decisions about their health and take timely actions to address any concerns.

By being proactive in seeking information online, individuals can take immediate steps to address health concerns, potentially avoiding unnecessary delays in seeking medical assistance. This proactive approach can also contribute to a sense of self-efficacy and enable individuals to take ownership of their health, thereby leading to more effective management of health-related issues.

Accessing reputable internet resources and e-books can also provide individuals with valuable insights into the best strategies for managing their health. Through targeted research, individuals can gain access to a wealth of information, including recommended treatment options, lifestyle modifications, and preventive measures. This access to diverse sources of information can empower individuals to make well-informed decisions about their health and take proactive steps to improve their overall well-being.

The use of internet resources for healthcare and self-care can have far-reaching implications for public health and governmental policies. By promoting access to reliable health information online, governments can facilitate the dissemination of vital health knowledge, thereby empowering individuals to make informed choices about their well-being. This can contribute to the creation of simple and safe pathways for people to access health information and resources, leading to a population that is better informed and more capable of taking charge of their own health.

In essence, by harnessing the power of the internet to research health-related topics and explore self-care strategies, individuals can play an active role in managing their well-being and making informed decisions about their health. This proactive approach not only maximizes the effective use of time but also fosters a sense of empowerment and self-responsibility. Additionally, the utilization of online resources for health and self-care has the potential to contribute to the creation of a more knowledgeable and self-sufficient society, ultimately leading to a life full of health freedom and well-being for individuals and communities alike.

Absolutely, taking charge of your health can indeed be empowering. By proactively seeking knowledge about healthcare and medical conditions on the internet, individuals can gain a better understanding of their own health and take more ownership of their well-being. Utilizing the abundance of online resources, including reputable websites, e-books, and medical journals, provides access to a wealth of information to make informed decisions about one's health. This proactive approach can help individuals make lifestyle changes, identify symptoms, and assess when professional medical assistance is necessary, potentially leading to early detection of health issues. However, it's essential to emphasize the importance of verifying information with credible sources and consulting with qualified healthcare professionals when needed.

Furthermore, this approach can lead to more efficient use of time as individuals can pursue information at their convenience and make informed decisions about their health without waiting for appointments or consultations with healthcare specialists. It allows individuals to be proactive in managing their health, potentially leading to earlier interventions and more effective treatment plans, ultimately saving time and potentially improving health outcomes.

Moreover, individuals using the internet to research health-related information can complement their understanding of medical conditions, treatment options, and preventive measures. This knowledge empowers individuals to engage in conversations with healthcare providers more effectively, fostering a collaborative approach to healthcare and promoting shared decision-making.

In addition, self-education through internet resources can contribute to overall societal health by promoting a more informed and engaged population. This, in turn, can support governments in developing public health initiatives and policies that are more aligned with the needs and concerns of the community. Access to reliable health information online can contribute to increased health literacy at a population level, leading to improved public health outcomes and reduced healthcare disparities.

However, it's essential to acknowledge potential pitfalls, such as misinformation, biased content, and the limitations of self-diagnosis and treatment. Encouraging individuals to approach online health information critically and seek professional guidance when necessary is crucial. Governments and public health authorities can play a role in promoting digital health literacy and ensuring the availability of accurate health information online, as well as regulating the quality of health-related content.

While leveraging internet resources for health-related information can empower individuals to take an active role in their health, it's crucial to balance self-education with professional guidance. By adopting a discerning and proactive approach to health information online, individuals can enhance their well-being, potentially contribute to improved public health, and find greater agency in managing their health.

Taking control of our health and well-being is a powerful step towards self-empowerment. By embracing the idea that we can help ourselves without always waiting for specialized medical professionals, we open the door to a world of possibilities. This shift in mindset allows us to use our time effectively, focusing on proactive health measures and self-care practices.

When we recognize that we can be our own best health advocates, we free ourselves from the constraints of traditional healthcare systems. By harnessing the vast knowledge available on the internet, we can educate ourselves about various health conditions, symptoms, and treatments. This self-education empowers us to make informed decisions about our health and well-being.

One of the key benefits of using the internet to research health-related topics is the access to a wide range of resources, including e-books and articles. By delving into these resources, we can learn about the latest medical advancements, holistic healing practices, and preventive care strategies. This knowledge equips us with the tools to create personalized health plans that suit our individual needs.

Through self-research and exploration, we can discover the best strategies for maintaining our health and preventing illnesses. By implementing these strategies into our daily routines, we take proactive steps towards a healthier lifestyle. This proactive approach not only benefits us individually but also contributes to a healthier community and society as a whole.

By embracing the role of being our own "doctor," we become more attuned to our bodies and health needs. We learn to listen to our bodies, recognize early warning signs, and take action to address any concerns promptly. This heightened self-awareness enables us to detect potential health issues early on, leading to better health outcomes in the long run.

By utilizing internet resources to empower ourselves in matters of health, we can help governments design simpler and safer healthcare initiatives. By promoting digital health literacy and self-care practices, governments can work towards creating a more informed and proactive population. This, in turn, can lead to reduced healthcare costs, improved public health, and a higher quality of life for all.

When individuals take charge of their health and well-being, it creates a ripple effect that extends beyond personal benefits. By living a life focused on health freedom, we inspire others to do the same. This collective shift towards self-care and self-empowerment can revolutionize the way society approaches healthcare, moving towards a more preventive and holistic model of wellness.

Embracing the idea of being our own doctors through internet research and self-care practices is a transformative journey towards health empowerment. By utilizing online resources, educating ourselves, and implementing personalized health strategies, we can take control of our well-being and lead healthier, more fulfilling lives. This proactive approach not only benefits us as individuals but also has the potential to shape a healthier and more empowered society for generations to come.

Certainly, self-care and taking charge of our health are important aspects of well-being. In today's digital age, the internet can be a valuable tool for individuals seeking to understand and address their health concerns. By empowering ourselves with knowledge and information, we can take proactive steps to improve our health and well-being without solely relying on healthcare professionals. Utilizing internet resources, such as reputable websites, medical journals, and e-books, can equip individuals with valuable insights and strategies to manage their health effectively.

By leveraging the power of the internet, individuals can access a wealth of information about various illnesses and conditions. This can enable individuals to make informed decisions about their health and well-being, leading to proactive measures in managing their conditions. Additionally, the internet can serve as a platform for individuals to connect with others who may be experiencing similar health challenges, fostering a sense of community and support.

Embracing a self-directed approach to health through internet research can lead to more efficient use of time and resources. Instead of waiting for appointments with specialized healthcare providers, individuals can take immediate action to understand and address their health concerns. This proactive approach can lead to early intervention and better health outcomes.

By encouraging individuals to be proactive in their health management, governments can also benefit from the positive impact of empowering citizens to be their own health advocates. This shift towards self-care and utilizing internet resources can alleviate the burden on healthcare systems, allowing for more effective allocation of resources and improved access to critical medical services for those in need.

Embracing a self-directed approach to health can lead to a sense of autonomy and empowerment among individuals. By taking an active role in their health and well-being, individuals can develop a deeper understanding of their bodies and health needs. This can ultimately lead to more holistic and personalized approaches to health management, fostering a strong sense of agency and self-advocacy.

In addition, leveraging internet resources for health research and self-care can also contribute to the democratization of health information. Individuals from diverse backgrounds and geographical locations can access valuable health insights and strategies, promoting a more inclusive approach to health and well-being. This can ultimately lead to more equitable access to health resources and information for individuals around the world.

Embracing self-care and utilizing internet resources for health management can contribute to the creation of a culture of prevention and proactive health maintenance. Through proactive measures such as regular health screenings, lifestyle modifications, and early intervention, individuals can work towards preventing illness and promoting long-term well-being. This can have far-reaching implications for public health and contribute to a more sustainable and resilient healthcare system.

By leveraging internet resources for health research and self-care, individuals can also develop a more comprehensive understanding of potential treatment options and complementary therapies. This can lead to more informed decision-making about their health, fostering a sense of empowerment and autonomy in their health journeys.

In summation, embracing a self-directed approach to health through internet research and self-care can have profound implications for individuals, communities, and governments. By empowering individuals with knowledge, strategies, and resources, the internet can serve as a powerful tool for promoting proactive health management and fostering a culture of well-being. This can ultimately lead to improved health outcomes, more efficient use of resources, and a more empowered and proactive approach to personal health and well-being.

Chapter Three: Empowering Health Freedom: Navigating Healthcare Challenges and Avoiding Medicine-Based Criminal Activities Through Self-Care and Internet Research

In today's evolving world, where healthcare systems worldwide face varying levels of challenges, there is a growing need for individuals to empower themselves in matters of health. The disparities in medical services, coupled with the potential risks of falling victim to medicine-based criminal activities, highlight the importance of taking charge of one's health. By proactively educating oneself and utilizing online resources, individuals can learn how to navigate health concerns effectively without solely relying on specialized medical professionals. This shift towards self-care not only promotes personal empowerment but also increases efficiency in managing health issues.

Accessing information on the internet has become a revolutionary way for individuals to stay informed about their health conditions. By conducting thorough research online, individuals can equip themselves with the necessary knowledge to make informed decisions about their well-being. Moreover, leveraging internet resources such as e-books can offer valuable insights into managing specific health issues and exploring alternative treatment options. This proactive approach not only fosters a sense of independence but also enables individuals to take control of their health journey.

Empowering individuals to become their own health advocates through internet research can lead to the development of effective strategies for managing health concerns. By tapping into a wealth of online information, individuals can explore various treatment approaches, preventive measures, and lifestyle interventions to address their unique health needs. This self-directed approach to healthcare enables individuals to tailor their strategies based on their research findings, preferences, and health goals. By leveraging these resources effectively, individuals can optimize their health outcomes and well-being.

The utilization of online platforms for health-related research and self-care not only benefits individuals but also contributes to broader public health initiatives. Governments can leverage the collective empowerment of individuals through internet-based health resources to promote preventive measures, public health education, and early intervention strategies. By creating simple and safe pathways for individuals to access reliable health information, governments can empower citizens to lead healthier lives and reduce the burden on formal healthcare systems. This collaborative effort between individuals and governing bodies paves the way for a society that prioritizes health freedom and individual empowerment.

As individuals take on a more active role in managing their health using online resources, they contribute to a paradigm shift in healthcare dynamics. By embracing the concept of being one's own doctor, individuals can proactively address health concerns, make informed decisions, and seek out solutions that align with their values and preferences. This shift towards self-care not only enhances individual autonomy but also fosters a culture of proactive health management and well-being. Through this approach, individuals can navigate the complexities of the healthcare system with greater confidence and agency.

The empowerment of individuals to become active participants in their health journey through internet research signifies a transformative approach to healthcare. By harnessing the vast array of health information available online, individuals can educate themselves on a wide range of health topics, conditions, and treatments. This knowledge empowerment enables individuals to make informed choices, advocate for their healthcare needs, and engage in meaningful discussions with healthcare providers. By embracing this proactive approach to health management, individuals can cultivate a deeper understanding of their well-being and take proactive steps towards achieving optimal health outcomes.

Transitioning towards a self-care model of health management through internet research can lead to improved health literacy and empowerment among individuals. By equipping individuals with the tools and resources to explore health information independently, they can make informed decisions about their health and well-being. This approach not only promotes self-sufficiency but also encourages individuals to engage in ongoing learning and exploration of health-related topics. By fostering a culture of continuous education and empowerment, individuals can develop a proactive stance towards health that prioritizes prevention, holistic well-being, and informed decision-making.

The integration of internet-based health resources into individual health management practices fosters a collaborative and proactive approach to healthcare. By utilizing these resources, individuals can access a wide range of information, tools, and support networks to navigate their health concerns effectively. This empowerment enables individuals to take a more active role in managing their health, seeking out relevant information, and exploring innovative health solutions. By engaging with online platforms, individuals can enhance their health knowledge, connect with like-minded individuals, and access personalized resources to support their unique health goals. This participatory approach not only enriches individual health journeys but also contributes to a collective culture of health empowerment and well-being.

The paradigm shift towards self-care and internet-based health management presents significant opportunities for individuals to optimize their health outcomes and well-being. By embracing a proactive approach to health through online research and resource utilization, individuals can cultivate a deeper understanding of their health concerns, treatment options, and preventive strategies. This transformative shift empowers individuals to become informed decision-makers, advocates for their health needs, and partners in their healthcare journey. By leveraging internet resources effectively, individuals can enhance their health literacy, improve their self-care practices, and take proactive steps towards achieving optimal health and well-being.

In the third chapter of a guide focused on avoiding medicine-based criminal activities, it's essential to emphasize proactive strategies individuals can employ when seeking healthcare services. When navigating health care centers, vigilance is key to prevent falling victim to potential scams or fraudulent practices. By taking ownership of one's health journey, individuals can empower themselves to make informed decisions while at the same time avoiding being misled by unscrupulous individuals posing as medical professionals. This proactive approach not only safeguards one's well-being but also contributes to the overall integrity of the healthcare system.

Empowering oneself with knowledge and information about common medical issues through reputable online sources can be a game-changer in self-care practices. By utilizing the vast resources available on the internet, individuals can equip themselves with reliable information on symptoms, treatments, and preventative measures. Moreover, conducting thorough research on one's health concerns can pave the way for effective communication with healthcare providers, facilitating a more collaborative approach towards personal well-being. This proactive engagement with online resources enables individuals to make well-informed decisions about their health without solely relying on external expertise.

Embracing the role of being one's own doctor through internet research can lead to significant benefits in terms of time management and self-care. Rather than waiting for specialized medical professionals for every minor health issue, individuals can leverage online platforms to gain insights into potential remedies and solutions. This approach not only enhances individual autonomy but also encourages a proactive attitude towards health maintenance and well-being. By taking charge of their health journey, individuals can optimize their time effectively and address medical concerns promptly without unnecessary delays.

Engaging with internet resources, such as e-books and online articles, can provide a wealth of knowledge on various health topics, enabling individuals to adopt best practices for self-care and wellness. Through continuous learning and self-education, individuals can broaden their understanding of health-related matters and develop practical strategies to maintain their well-being. This digital empowerment not only enhances individual autonomy but also promotes a culture of self-sufficiency and proactive health management. By utilizing online resources wisely, individuals can navigate the complexities of healthcare with confidence and make informed decisions about their health and wellness.

The shift towards individuals taking a more active role in their healthcare through internet research has broader societal implications, including potential benefits for governments in promoting public health initiatives. By encouraging citizens to leverage online resources for self-care and medical information, governments can foster a culture of health literacy and empower individuals to make informed choices about their well-being. This, in turn, can lead to the development of streamlined and accessible healthcare policies that prioritize preventive care and patient education. Governments that support and promote the use of internet resources for health management can enhance the overall well-being of their populations and create a healthcare system that is both efficient and patient-centered.

By embracing the idea of being one's own doctor through internet research, individuals not only empower themselves to make well-informed decisions about their health but also contribute to the larger goal of promoting health freedom and autonomy. Through proactive engagement with online resources and a commitment to self-education, individuals can take control of their health journey and navigate healthcare systems with confidence and efficacy. This shift towards self-care and digital empowerment signifies a transformative approach to personal well-being, wherein individuals become active participants in their health management and advocate for a healthcare system that prioritizes transparency, accessibility, and patient empowerment. In essence, by leveraging internet resources for health-related information and self-care practices, individuals can pave the way for a future where everyone has the tools and knowledge to lead a healthy, fulfilling life.

In today's modern world, where medical crimes and unethical practices can sometimes lurk within healthcare centers, it is imperative for individuals to take charge of their health and well-being. By arming ourselves with knowledge and not solely relying on specialized professionals, we can navigate the intricacies of the healthcare system more efficiently. This proactive approach allows us to save time and energy by being self-sufficient and self-caring in our health endeavors. Embracing the role of one's own doctor through the vast resources available on the internet empowers individuals to make informed decisions about their health.

When a person delves into researching their health concerns online, they unlock a treasure trove of information that can guide them in implementing the best strategies for their well-being. The internet provides a platform for accessing e-books, articles, and reputable sources that can significantly enhance one's understanding of various health conditions. This wealth of knowledge not only aids in self-diagnosis but also equips individuals with the tools to take proactive measures towards their health maintenance.

The utilization of internet resources in managing one's health can extend beyond personal benefits. Governments can leverage the power of digital platforms to create simple and secure healthcare solutions for the public. By promoting the dissemination of accurate health information online, governments can facilitate a society that embraces health freedom and wellness. This shift towards accessible healthcare through the internet can revolutionize the way individuals interact with the healthcare system.

Embracing the concept of being one's own doctor through online resources is not about replacing medical professionals but about supplementing traditional healthcare practices with self-empowerment and knowledge. Through adopting a proactive stance towards health management, individuals can proactively prevent illnesses, monitor their well-being effectively, and make informed decisions about their healthcare. By bridging the gap between medical expertise and personal responsibility, individuals can navigate the complex landscape of healthcare with confidence and autonomy.

The empowerment that comes from being one's own health advocate extends beyond the confines of traditional healthcare settings. By utilizing internet resources for health-related research, individuals can tap into a vast pool of information that was once inaccessible. This democratization of healthcare knowledge breaks down barriers to understanding and allows individuals to take control of their health outcomes. In a world where information is power, being well-informed about one's health can be a transformative tool for personal wellness and longevity.

The ability to access e-books, webinars, and credible health websites enables individuals to delve deeper into specific health topics and strategies. With just a few clicks, individuals can educate themselves on preventive measures, treatment options, and holistic approaches to well-being. This empowerment through knowledge not only enhances personal health but also promotes a culture of proactive self-care and wellness within communities.

By embracing the role of one's own doctor through internet research and resource utilization, individuals can navigate the healthcare landscape with confidence and efficacy. This shift towards self-empowerment in health management fosters a sense of responsibility and agency in individuals, allowing them to make informed decisions about their well-being. By leveraging the wealth of information available online, individuals can proactively engage in their health journey and promote a culture of self-care and wellness.

The transformative potential of internet-based health research extends beyond individual empowerment to societal impact. By encouraging individuals to take charge of their health through digital resources, governments can pave the way for a healthier population. By leveraging technology to disseminate accurate health information, governments can create avenues for preventive healthcare, early intervention, and comprehensive wellness strategies. This collaboration between individuals, technology, and governments can revolutionize the healthcare landscape and lead to a society that prioritizes health freedom and well-being.

The paradigm shift towards being one's own doctor through internet-based research represents a transformative approach to healthcare. By embracing the wealth of information available online, individuals can proactively engage in their health journey, make informed decisions, and promote a culture of empowerment and wellness. This self-care mindset not only benefits individuals but also has the potential to revolutionize the healthcare system, creating a society that values health freedom, autonomy, and proactive well-being.

In a world where healthcare can sometimes be daunting due to potential risks of medicine-based criminal activities, empowering yourself with knowledge and utilizing the resources available on the internet can be a game-changer. Rather than solely depending on traditional healthcare centers and specialists, taking proactive steps to be your own health advocate can lead to more effective and efficient self-care practices. By taking the initiative to research your own health concerns online, you can equip yourself with information that empowers you to make informed decisions regarding your well-being.

The accessibility of the internet allows individuals to take charge of their health by utilizing a wealth of resources at their fingertips. Engaging in research about illnesses and health conditions can not only enhance your understanding but also provide insight into various treatment options, preventive measures, and lifestyle changes. Through online platforms, individuals can access a wide array of reliable information, including e-books, articles, and reputable websites that offer valuable insights into health and wellness.

By leveraging the power of the internet, individuals can adopt best strategies for managing their health effectively. From learning about alternative remedies to understanding potential side effects of certain medications, the online world opens up a myriad of possibilities for individuals to customize their health approach. Moreover, by exploring e-books and other digital resources, individuals can delve deeper into specific health topics, gaining a comprehensive understanding of their conditions and possible treatment pathways.

Taking a proactive approach to one's health not only benefits individuals but also has broader implications for societal health and well-being. As more people embrace self-care practices and empower themselves with knowledge, it propels governments to develop simple and secure avenues for individuals to access healthcare information and services. By promoting a culture of health literacy and self-advocacy, governments can foster a society where individuals are actively engaged in their well-being and can make informed choices that contribute to a healthier, more empowered population.

Through self-education and utilizing internet resources, individuals can break free from the dependency on traditional healthcare systems and effectively become their own doctors in many aspects. The internet serves as a platform where individuals can explore various perspectives, treatments, and expert opinions, allowing them to tailor their healthcare approach based on their unique needs and preferences. This shift towards self-care not only encourages personal responsibility but also promotes a proactive mindset that values preventive healthcare and holistic well-being.

Incorporating internet resources into one's health journey can revolutionize the way individuals monitor, manage, and enhance their well-being. Whether through online forums, telemedicine platforms, or informational websites, the internet offers a diverse range of tools that enable individuals to stay informed, connected, and empowered in their health decisions. By tapping into these resources, individuals can enhance their health literacy, engage in meaningful discussions with peers, and explore innovative solutions that align with their wellness goals.

By embracing the role of being one's own health advocate, individuals can navigate the complexities of the healthcare system with confidence and autonomy. Through active participation in their health management, individuals can stay ahead of potential risks, identify early warning signs, and take prompt action to address any health concerns. Empowering individuals to become proactive stewards of their health not only contributes to personal well-being but also fosters a culture of resilience and self-sufficiency that benefits society as a whole.

The shift towards embracing internet resources for self-care and health management represents a transformation in how individuals approach their well-being. By leveraging online tools for research, information gathering, and remote consultations, individuals can bridge gaps in healthcare access, improve health outcomes, and take control of their health destiny. This proactive mindset not only empowers individuals to make informed choices but also encourages a paradigm shift towards a more patient-centered, technology-enabled healthcare landscape.

The integration of internet resources into health management practices offers a transformative approach to wellness that empowers individuals to take charge of their health journey. By embracing the abundance of information, support networks, and digital tools available online, individuals can adopt a proactive stance towards their well-being, enhance their health literacy, and make informed decisions that prioritize long-term health and vitality. Through self-education, self-care, and self-advocacy, individuals can harness the power of the internet to lead healthier, more empowered lives while contributing to a society that values health freedom and personal responsibility.

Healthcare is a crucial aspect of every individual's life, and navigating the complexities of medical treatment can be challenging. When seeking medical help, it's vital to be aware of potential criminal activities related to medications and healthcare practices. Educating oneself about potential pitfalls and red flags is crucial. By being well-informed about the proper usage of medications and understanding potential risks of misuse or criminal activities, individuals can protect themselves from falling victim to illegal practices. This self-awareness and understanding of medication-related criminal activities can help individuals make informed decisions about their healthcare and avoid potential harm.

In today's fast-paced world, time is a valuable asset, and waiting for specialized medical professionals may not always be viable. Utilizing internet resources to empower oneself with knowledge about healthcare and understanding potential treatments can be an effective way to take control of one's health. Internet-based research can lead to valuable insights and understanding, enabling individuals to make informed decisions about their health and well-being. By utilizing time effectively and being proactive in self-care, individuals can take charge of their health and well-being, minimizing the need for excessive reliance on traditional healthcare systems.

Access to information and resources on the internet can empower individuals to take charge of their health effectively. Through careful research on reputable websites and leveraging online resources such as e-books, individuals can broaden their understanding of various health conditions and treatment options. This can enable individuals to make informed choices about their health and explore alternative or complementary therapies. By embracing the opportunity to become their own health advocate, individuals can take proactive steps towards maintaining their well-being and making informed decisions about healthcare.

Incorporating internet-based strategies into healthcare can also have broader implications for society. Governments can leverage the power of online resources to create simple and safe avenues for people to access reliable health information. By promoting access to credible health resources, governments can empower individuals to lead healthier lives and make informed decisions about their well-being. This approach can contribute to fostering a society that values health freedom and empowers individuals to take proactive steps towards maintaining their well-being.

By harnessing the wealth of reliable information available on the internet, individuals can equip themselves with the knowledge and understanding to navigate the complexities of healthcare. This proactive approach to self-education and empowerment can help individuals avoid falling victim to potential medication-based criminal activities and make informed decisions about their health. Embracing the opportunities presented by internet resources and promoting self-care can lead to a society that values health freedom and empowers individuals to take proactive steps towards maintaining their well-being.

It is increasingly essential to recognize the potential risks associated with medicine-based criminal activities within healthcare settings. Understanding and being aware of these risks can empower individuals to take proactive measures to safeguard themselves. By proactively engaging in self-care and leveraging readily available resources, individuals can significantly mitigate the risks associated with potential medicine-based criminal activities. This includes being educated about their health, utilizing reliable internet resources, and adopting a preventive approach to wellness.

Empowering oneself with knowledge and being proactive about healthcare can lead to a more efficient use of time. Instead of relying solely on specialized healthcare professionals, individuals can take charge of their own well-being. This shift in approach not only leads to personal empowerment but also contributes to a more effective utilization of healthcare resources.

Utilizing internet resources to conduct research on health-related matters provides individuals with the opportunity to delve into various strategies and gain insights into potential treatment options. Accessing e-books and informative articles can offer valuable knowledge and guidance, allowing individuals to make informed decisions about their health. This approach facilitates a sense of self-sufficiency and independence in managing one's well-being.

The proactive engagement in self-care and leveraging of internet resources can have broader societal implications. It can lead to a more informed populace that is actively involved in their health management. This, in turn, can influence governments to develop simple and secure channels for individuals to access healthcare information and resources. By promoting a culture of self-care and empowerment, governments can contribute to creating a society that values health freedom and individual responsibility for well-being.

Taking charge of one's health through internet-based resources can also serve as a form of prevention against potential medicine-based criminal activities. By educating oneself and implementing preventive strategies, individuals can reduce their vulnerability to fraudulent schemes and unauthorized medical interventions. This proactive stance not only benefits individuals but also contributes to the overall integrity of healthcare systems and the protection of public health.

In conclusion, the proactive adoption of self-care practices and the utilization of internet resources can significantly reduce the risks associated with potential medicine-based criminal activities in healthcare settings. Embracing a mentality of self-responsibility for health, leveraging accessible information, and advocating for health freedom can have profound implications for individuals and society as a whole. It is through proactive education, self-empowerment, and informed decision-making that individuals can navigate the complexities of healthcare with resilience and confidence.

Chapter Four: Empowering Self-Care: A Path to Health Freedom and Legal Recognition

In today's rapidly advancing world, the legal recognition of self-care practices within the healthcare landscape is essential. Governments play a pivotal role in this endeavor, as they can provide the necessary legal framework to empower individuals to take charge of their health without being subjected to potential criminal activities linked to unregulated medicine. This proactive approach allows individuals to seek treatment and wellness on their own terms, avoiding unnecessary waiting times and delays by not solely relying on specialized medical professionals. Accessing reputable internet resources becomes a valuable tool in this journey towards self-care, allowing individuals to educate themselves and make informed decisions about their health.

By acknowledging the significance of internet-based research, individuals can harness the wealth of knowledge available online, enabling them to adopt effective self-care strategies. This includes the utilization of e-books and other digital resources that offer comprehensive insights into various health concerns. Moreover, the integration of such practices can also benefit governments by facilitating the creation of user-friendly and secure platforms that streamline access to reliable health information. Establishing simplified pathways to health and well-being promotes a sense of freedom and autonomy within communities, ultimately contributing to a society where individuals are empowered to lead healthier and more fulfilling lives.

Legal recognition of self-care as a valid and effective healthcare approach can serve as a transformative catalyst for individuals and societies alike. It facilitates a paradigm shift towards a more proactive and preventative approach to health, diminishing the reliance on traditional healthcare systems for every minor ailment or concern. Embracing self-care not only grants individuals the autonomy to address their health needs promptly but also fosters a deeper sense of responsibility and empowerment. By advocating for legal avenues that endorse self-care, governments can pave the way for a more equitable and accessible healthcare landscape, with individuals equipped to navigate their health journey with confidence and competence.

Acknowledging the pivotal role of the internet in enabling self-care is paramount. Through comprehensive research and exploration of trusted online resources, individuals can equip themselves with a diverse array of health-related knowledge, enabling them to make informed decisions about their well-being. This dynamic utilization of technology empowers individuals to be proactive in managing their health, ultimately reducing the burden on traditional healthcare systems and ensuring timely access to essential information and support.

At its core, legal recognition of self-care and the facilitation of internet-driven health literacy present governments with a unique opportunity to foster a culture of well-being and empowerment. By embracing these concepts, individuals can navigate their health journeys with confidence, leveraging the vast resources available online to make informed decisions and pursue optimal health outcomes. This paradigm shift not only bolsters individual autonomy but also supports the broader goal of promoting public health and well-being, ultimately leading to healthier, more engaged communities.

Legal recognition of alternative methods of healthcare, such as self-care and internet-based resources, has the potential to significantly impact individuals' access to medical information and empower them to take control of their health. By granting legal recognition to these non-traditional forms of healthcare, governments can help mitigate the risks associated with unregulated medical practices and provide individuals with the tools to make informed decisions about their health.

One of the primary benefits of legal recognition for alternative healthcare methods is the potential to reduce the prevalence of medicine-based criminal activities. By legitimizing non-traditional approaches to healthcare, individuals may be less inclined to seek out unlicensed or illicit medical treatments, thereby decreasing the opportunity for criminal exploitation within the healthcare industry.

Legal recognition of self-care and internet-based healthcare resources can promote efficiency in healthcare utilization. Individuals can access medical information and resources promptly, without having to wait for specialized medical professionals. This empowerment can lead to more timely and proactive management of health concerns, potentially reducing the burden on traditional healthcare systems.

Recognizing self-care and internet-based healthcare resources can encourage individuals to take greater responsibility for their own health and well-being. Through access to credible online resources and e-books, individuals can educate themselves about various health conditions, treatment options, and preventive measures. This knowledge empowers individuals to make informed decisions about their health, promoting a proactive and self-directed approach to wellness.

Additionally, by embracing these alternative healthcare modalities, governments can contribute to the creation of simple and secure pathways for individuals to lead healthier lives. Legal recognition can enable the development of regulatory frameworks that ensure the quality and safety of internet-based healthcare resources, offering individuals reliable and trustworthy platforms for self-care and health management.

Recognizing the value of self-care and internet-based healthcare resources can also serve as a catalyst for promoting health freedom. Individuals may feel more empowered to explore diverse healthcare options, customize their wellness strategies, and pursue treatments that align with their personal beliefs and preferences. This freedom to choose can lead to greater satisfaction and confidence in healthcare decision-making.

Overall, legal recognition of alternative healthcare methods can potentially foster a shift towards a more holistic and inclusive approach to healthcare. By acknowledging the validity and effectiveness of self-care and internet-based resources, governments can support diverse healthcare choices and promote a sense of agency and autonomy among individuals in managing their health.

The legal recognition of self-care and internet-based healthcare resources has the potential to mitigate medicine-based criminal activities, promote efficiency in healthcare utilization, encourage individual responsibility for health, and contribute to the creation of simple and safe pathways for health management. Additionally, it can foster health freedom, allowing individuals to lead healthier lives with access to a wide range of healthcare options. Recognizing the value of these alternative healthcare modalities presents an opportunity for governments to support a more inclusive and proactive approach to healthcare, ultimately benefiting individuals and communities as a whole.

Legal recognition of individuals taking control of their health without solely relying on traditional medicine is a progressive step towards empowering individuals to be proactive in managing their own well-being. Governments play a crucial role in endorsing this concept by acknowledging and legitimizing the use of alternative health practices and self-care methods. By granting legal recognition to such practices, governments can establish frameworks that protect individuals from potential criminal activities within the healthcare sector. This recognition can also pave the way for individuals to seek out alternative solutions without fear of repercussions, thereby promoting a more holistic approach to healthcare.

In many cases, individuals may encounter fraudulent or criminal activities within the realm of traditional medicine, such as counterfeit medications or unauthorized treatments. By legally recognizing alternative health practices and self-care methods, governments can mitigate the risks associated with such criminal acts, offering individuals a safer and more transparent healthcare environment. This recognition can provide individuals with the confidence to explore alternative avenues for their health and well-being, without the need to solely rely on traditional medical establishments.

Empowering individuals to take charge of their health through self-care and alternative health practices not only saves time but also enables individuals to be more proactive in their well-being. By utilizing resources available on the internet, individuals can educate themselves about various health conditions, treatments, and self-care techniques. This knowledge empowers individuals to make informed decisions about their health and explore alternative solutions that align with their preferences and values.

Researching one's health condition on the internet can equip individuals with valuable insights and information to make informed choices about their well-being. By leveraging internet resources, such as e-books, articles, and online forums, individuals can access a wealth of information to better understand their health conditions and explore alternative treatment options. This self-education can empower individuals to take a more active role in managing their health and well-being, leading to greater autonomy and control over their healthcare decisions.

Encouraging individuals to become their own health advocates and doctors by utilizing internet resources can revolutionize the way people approach their wellness. By leveraging the vast information available online, individuals can access a wide range of perspectives, treatment options, and self-care techniques that may not be readily available within traditional healthcare settings. This shift towards self-care and self-education promotes a proactive approach to health and well-being, fostering a culture of empowered and informed individuals who take responsibility for their own health outcomes.

Legal recognition of individuals using the internet as a tool for self-care can also benefit governments by promoting health literacy and prevention strategies among the population. By encouraging individuals to explore alternative health solutions online, governments can support initiatives that prioritize preventive care, early intervention, and lifestyle modifications. This proactive approach to healthcare not only empowers individuals to make healthier choices but also reduces the burden on traditional healthcare systems by promoting preventive measures and self-management strategies.

The embrace of self-care and alternative health practices through internet research can open doors to a more inclusive and diverse healthcare landscape. By recognizing individuals' rights to explore alternative health solutions and make informed decisions about their well-being, governments can foster a healthcare system that values individual autonomy and choice. This diversity in healthcare options not only promotes innovation and personalized care but also creates a more patient-centered approach to wellness that prioritizes individual preferences and needs.

Governments can play a pivotal role in creating simple and safe pathways for individuals to access alternative health practices and self-care methods through online channels. By establishing guidelines, regulations, and support systems for individuals seeking alternative health solutions, governments can ensure that individuals have access to reliable and credible information to make informed decisions about their health. This supportive environment can encourage individuals to take a more active role in their well-being and explore alternative avenues for healthcare that resonate with their beliefs and values.

Legal recognition of individuals being their own doctors through internet research can contribute to a culture of health freedom and personal empowerment. By endorsing individuals' autonomy in making healthcare decisions and exploring alternative health practices, governments can promote a sense of empowerment and self-reliance among the population. This shift towards health freedom encourages individuals to take ownership of their health outcomes, make informed choices, and prioritize self-care, ultimately leading to a society that values individual agency and well-being.

Legal recognition of individuals taking control of their health through self-care and internet research is a transformative step towards creating a healthcare system that prioritizes individual empowerment, safety, and well-being. By endorsing alternative health practices, promoting self-care strategies, and supporting individuals in making informed decisions about their health, governments can facilitate a cultural shift towards a more empowered, proactive, and health-conscious society. Embracing self-care, internet research, and alternative health solutions can pave the way for a future where individuals have the knowledge, resources, and autonomy to lead healthy and fulfilling lives.

The fourth chapter will emphasize how governments should legally recognize and support individuals taking charge of their own health, without depending solely on traditional medicine or healthcare professionals. By providing legal recognition, governments can establish frameworks that empower individuals to take responsibility for their health and well-being. This legal recognition would offer protection against any potential criminal repercussions individuals might face when seeking alternative health solutions outside of traditional medicine. It would also promote the utilization of internet resources and self-care practices, allowing individuals to make informed health decisions and utilize their time effectively.

Legal recognition of self-care and alternative health practices can ensure that individuals are not subjected to criminal implications when seeking non-traditional health solutions. By providing a legal framework for these practices, governments can cultivate an environment where individuals feel supported in their pursuit of alternative healthcare methods, thereby encouraging them to take proactive measures for their well-being.

Legal recognition can aid in the establishment of comprehensive guidelines and best practices for individuals conducting research on their health issues using internet resources. This can include accessing reputable e-books and online materials to develop a deep understanding of their conditions. Encouraging individuals to leverage internet resources for health-related research can lead to the adoption of best strategies and practices, thereby promoting informed decision-making in self-care.

Chapter Five: Empowering Health Freedom: Liberating Individuals through Knowledge and Autonomy

In this chapter, we delve into the critical importance of securing human freedom within the realm of healthcare, a sphere often intertwined with legal regulations imposed by governments. Ensuring individuals have the right to make informed decisions about their health can be a pivotal step in thwarting potential criminal activities revolving around medicinal practices within the healthcare system. By advocating for autonomy in health choices, individuals can navigate the complexities of medical care without undue reliance on specialists, thereby optimizing their time and promoting self-care practices.

Moreover, harnessing the wealth of information available on the internet empowers individuals to take control of their health outcomes. Through diligent research on their conditions, individuals can equip themselves with valuable insights and strategic approaches to managing their health utilizing various online resources, including e-books. This shift towards self-education not only fosters personal empowerment but also presents an opportunity for governments to streamline healthcare processes, facilitating safer and more accessible ways for individuals to lead healthy lives free from undue restrictions.

By embracing the concept of being one's own doctor in the digital age, individuals can forge a path towards a healthier and more self-reliant future. The ability to leverage internet resources for medical research and guidance opens up a world of possibilities for informed decision-making and proactive health management. As individuals become more adept at utilizing online tools for health-related purposes, they not only enhance their own well-being but also contribute to the broader goal of promoting health freedom within society.

This newfound emphasis on individual agency in healthcare catalyzes a shift towards a more proactive and preventive approach to well-being. By encouraging individuals to be proactive in monitoring and addressing their health concerns, we lay the groundwork for a population that is not only healthier but also more resilient to potential health challenges. As individuals take charge of their health destiny through informed choices and digital empowerment, they contribute towards shaping a society that values personal autonomy and holistic well-being.

The convergence of technology and self-care practices offers a promising avenue for individuals to reclaim agency over their health journeys. Through access to a plethora of online resources and informational tools, individuals can transcend traditional barriers to healthcare and forge a path towards a more self-directed and empowering approach to well-being. This shift towards digital empowerment in healthcare not only benefits individuals but also paves the way for a more inclusive and accessible health system that prioritizes individual freedoms and well-being.

The quest for health freedom and autonomy is not just a personal endeavor but a collective aspiration with far-reaching implications. By advocating for individual empowerment in healthcare decisions, we pave the way for a society that values informed choices, self-care practices, and digital empowerment. As individuals embrace their role as active participants in their health journeys, they not only enhance their well-being but also contribute towards a healthier, more resilient society where health freedom is a fundamental right rather than a distant ideal.

By recognizing the value of self-care and the responsible utilization of internet resources, governments can facilitate the creation of simple and safe pathways for individuals to access alternative health solutions. This recognition can also enable the development of educational initiatives to guide individuals in utilizing internet resources to make informed health decisions, thereby promoting a life of health freedom.

In addition, legal recognition can serve as a catalyst for governments to collaborate with experts in alternative medicine, holistic health, and internet-based healthcare platforms. This collaboration can lead to the development of safe and effective guidelines for individuals to adopt self-care practices and make well-informed health decisions. By engaging with experts in the field, governments can ensure that the self-care framework is rooted in evidence-based practices and prioritizes the well-being of individuals.

Legal recognition can help in the establishment of safeguards that protect individuals from potential exploitation or misinformation when utilizing internet resources for self-care. This recognition can enable the implementation of regulatory measures to identify and mitigate fraudulent health information, thereby promoting a safe and reliable environment for individuals to navigate and utilize the internet for health-related purposes effectively.

Legal recognition can encourage the integration of self-care and internet-based health practices into the broader healthcare system. This integration can lead to the development of complementary healthcare pathways that allow individuals to seamlessly blend traditional and alternative health solutions. By embracing a holistic approach to healthcare, governments can facilitate a more inclusive and diverse healthcare landscape, empowering individuals to make informed decisions about their well-being.

Legal recognition of internet-based self-care practices can contribute to the democratization of health information. Through legal frameworks, governments can support initiatives that promote the accessibility of reliable health-related content on the internet, ultimately empowering individuals to access valuable resources and make informed decisions about their health. This shift towards democratizing health information can pave the way for a more inclusive and equitable healthcare ecosystem, where individuals have the tools and knowledge to actively participate in their own well-being.

By providing legal recognition and support for self-care, internet-based health research, and alternative health practices, governments can foster an environment where individuals are empowered to take charge of their health effectively. This legal recognition can serve as a cornerstone for promoting health freedom, protecting individuals from potential criminal repercussions, and establishing safe and accessible pathways for individuals to pursue alternative health solutions. Moreover, it can contribute to the development of a holistic healthcare landscape, where individuals have the autonomy and resources to make well-informed decisions about their well-being.

Acknowledging and legally recognizing the potential for individuals to take more responsibility for their health could revolutionize how we approach medical care. By granting legal recognition to self-care practices and empowering individuals to be proactive in maintaining their well-being, governments can help prevent instances of criminal activities related to the misuse or distribution of medications. This shift in perspective encourages people to take charge of their health rather than solely relying on healthcare professionals, ultimately leading to a more efficient use of time and resources. Through leveraging the vast information available on the internet, individuals can educate themselves about their health conditions and make informed decisions about their care, potentially reducing the burden on traditional healthcare systems.

It is crucial to emphasize the importance of self-education and empowerment in healthcare. When individuals have the tools and knowledge to research their health concerns online, they can discover effective strategies and treatment options that may not have been readily available to them otherwise. By utilizing resources such as e-books and reputable websites, individuals can access a wealth of information that can empower them to make informed choices about their health. Encouraging this self-directed approach to healthcare not only benefits individuals but also contributes to a more knowledgeable and health-conscious society.

Recognizing the role of self-care and self-education in healthcare can also lead to the development of simpler and safer healthcare pathways for individuals. By promoting a culture of self-care and empowering individuals to take control of their health, governments can create systems that prioritize prevention and wellness. This approach may help reduce the prevalence of preventable diseases and alleviate the strain on healthcare systems, resulting in a population that is healthier and more self-sufficient in managing their well-being. Furthermore, providing legal recognition and support for self-care practices can empower individuals to make informed decisions about their health without fear of legal repercussions, fostering a sense of autonomy and responsibility.

Empowering individuals to be their own advocates in healthcare can have far-reaching benefits for both individuals and society as a whole. By encouraging people to research their health concerns and explore alternative treatments, governments can promote a culture of wellness and self-reliance. This shift in mindset can lead to a decrease in unnecessary medical interventions, medication misuse, and healthcare fraud, ultimately contributing to a more sustainable and efficient healthcare system. Legal recognition of self-care practices can pave the way for innovative healthcare solutions that prioritize holistic well-being and individual empowerment.

Incorporating self-care practices into healthcare systems can fundamentally transform the way we approach health and wellness. By elevating the status of self-care and self-education, governments can empower individuals to make more informed decisions about their health and well-being. This proactive approach to healthcare not only enhances individual autonomy but also cultivates a sense of responsibility and empowerment among the population. Legal recognition of self-care practices can signal a paradigm shift in healthcare towards a more patient-centered and preventative model, fostering a culture of wellness and self-sufficiency.

Encouraging individuals to take a proactive approach to their health can lead to a multitude of positive outcomes. By empowering people to research their health concerns and explore alternative treatments, governments can promote a sense of personal agency and responsibility. This shift in mindset can help individuals avoid falling victim to misinformation or fraudulent practices in the healthcare system, ultimately leading to better health outcomes and a more educated populace. Legal recognition of self-care practices can serve as a catalyst for a more patient-centered and empowered approach to healthcare, paving the way for a healthier and more informed society.

Promoting self-care and self-education in healthcare can foster a culture of empowerment and well-being. By acknowledging the value of individuals taking control of their health and making informed decisions, governments can create a more resilient and proactive population. Embracing self-care practices can help reduce the burden on traditional healthcare systems, empower individuals to explore personalized wellness strategies, and promote a sense of ownership over one's health. Legal recognition of self-care practices can provide a strong foundation for a healthcare system that values prevention, education, and individual empowerment.

Empowering individuals to become their own healthcare advocates can lead to significant improvements in overall health outcomes. By encouraging people to research their health concerns and explore self-care options, governments can foster a culture of proactive and informed decision-making. This shift towards patient empowerment not only enhances individual well-being but also contributes to a more sustainable and efficient healthcare system. Legal recognition of self-care practices can lay the groundwork for a healthcare system that prioritizes prevention, education, and individual responsibility, ultimately leading to healthier and more self-sufficient communities.

By providing legal recognition and support for self-care practices, governments can help individuals navigate the complexities of the healthcare system with confidence and autonomy. Empowering people to take charge of their health and well-being through self-education and proactive measures can lead to a more efficient use of healthcare resources and a decrease in preventable illnesses. By leveraging the wealth of information available on the internet, individuals can access a variety of resources to better understand their health concerns and make informed decisions. This can lead to a more educated and health-conscious society, ultimately improving overall well-being and reducing the reliance on traditional medical interventions.

It is important to emphasize the critical role of assuring human freedom when governments give it legal recognition, particularly in the context of healthcare and medicine. When individuals are granted the freedom to take charge of their own health and well-being, it not only empowers them to make informed decisions but also significantly reduces the likelihood of falling victim to medicine-based criminal activities that may be prevalent in healthcare centers elsewhere. The legal recognition of this freedom not only fosters a sense of self-reliance but also enables individuals to utilize their time effectively, without necessarily having to wait for specialized medical professionals. This, in turn, promotes a culture of self-care that is not only personally empowering but also contributes to the overall wellbeing of the individual, thus positively impacting society as a whole.

In embracing the freedom to be one's own doctor – or at the very least, an informed and proactive partner in one's own healthcare journey – individuals are increasingly turning to the vast resources available on the internet. By conducting research on their illnesses and potential treatment options, individuals can harness the power of the internet to equip themselves with the best possible strategies for managing their health concerns. Additionally, the availability of e-books and other online resources further enhances the individual's capacity to become more knowledgeable and capable in addressing their health needs. It's crucial to recognize that this shift towards self-education and empowerment in healthcare not only benefits the individuals but also presents opportunities for governments to develop simplified and secure pathways that support people in living lives filled with health freedom.

This evolving trend not only gives recognition to the right of individuals to actively engage in their own healthcare decisions but also underscores the broader significance of health freedom within society. By leveraging the wealth of information available on the internet, individuals can gain a deeper understanding of their health conditions, potential treatments, and preventive measures, leading to more informed and proactive choices. Furthermore, the ability to access and understand health-related information online empowers individuals to make sound decisions that contribute to their overall wellness, reducing their susceptibility to misinformation and potential exploitation in healthcare settings. This increased individual autonomy in healthcare, when recognized and supported by governments, has the potential to foster a culture of self-advocacy and health consciousness, thereby promoting a society in which individuals are more equipped to protect and prioritize their own health and well-being.

By embracing the freedom to take charge of their health through internet-based resources, individuals can contribute to the creation of a more informed and health-conscious society. This heightened level of awareness and autonomy not only benefits the individuals themselves but also has wider implications for public health. As individuals become more knowledgeable about their health and healthcare options, they can make better decisions that lead to improved overall health outcomes. Additionally, the collective impact of individuals actively engaging in their own healthcare can significantly alleviate the burden on healthcare systems, allowing for more efficient allocation of resources and focused attention on critical cases. Recognizing and facilitating this self-empowerment in healthcare is therefore not only advantageous for individuals but also contributes to the broader societal goal of promoting health and wellness.

The legal recognition of the freedom to engage with healthcare independently through online resources can encourage the development of innovative and user-friendly initiatives by governments to promote health literacy and responsible self-care. Such initiatives can include the creation of accessible online platforms, educational tools, and reliable digital resources that enable individuals to navigate and understand health-related information effectively. In doing so, governments can play a pivotal role in facilitating a culture of informed decision-making and self-reliance in healthcare, ultimately contributing to a society where individuals are more empowered and capable of safeguarding their own health and well-being. Additionally, by embracing and supporting the concept of individuals being proactive in their healthcare, governments can foster a collaborative approach to health management, wherein individuals are encouraged to take ownership of their health while remaining supported by accessible and trustworthy resources and guidance. This collaborative approach not only strengthens individual agency in healthcare but also establishes a foundation for a more resilient and self-sufficient healthcare ecosystem within society.

It is imperative to recognize that the legal recognition of human freedom in healthcare, particularly in the context of utilizing internet resources, presents an opportunity for governments to create and implement policies that support individuals in living healthy and informed lives. By acknowledging and upholding this fundamental freedom, governments can proactively shape the healthcare landscape to be more inclusive, transparent, and conducive to individual empowerment. Through the establishment of comprehensive guidelines, regulatory frameworks, and educational initiatives, governments can play a pivotal role in promoting a culture of health freedom that encourages individuals to actively participate in their own healthcare journeys, leveraging internet-based resources to make informed decisions and manage their well-being effectively. This approach not only aligns with the principles of personal autonomy and responsibility but also holds the potential to significantly enhance public health outcomes and contribute to the overall well-being of society at large.

When governments legally recognize and assure human freedom in healthcare, they empower individuals to take charge of their health and well-being. This acknowledgment signifies an essential shift towards a more patient-centered approach, emphasizing autonomy and self-determination. By providing legal recognition to human freedom in healthcare, governments not only affirm the fundamental rights of individuals but also inspire a sense of responsibility and empowerment.

Legal recognition of human freedom in healthcare is crucial for preventing medicine-based criminal activities that individuals may face when seeking medical assistance. By promoting access to accurate and reliable health information and resources, governments can mitigate the risks associated with fraudulent or illicit medical practices. This not only protects individuals from potential harm but also fosters a climate of trust and transparency within the healthcare system.

Empowering individuals to take a proactive role in their healthcare can yield substantial benefits in terms of time management and resource utilization. By leveraging internet-based resources and information, individuals can educate themselves about various health conditions, treatment options, and preventive measures. This autonomy enables them to make informed decisions and manage their health effectively, without solely relying on specialized medical professionals.

The utilization of internet resources for self-care not only enables individuals to be more independent but also facilitates greater efficiency in managing their health. With access to a plethora of reputable health websites, online forums, and digital healthcare platforms, individuals can harness the power of information to address their health concerns promptly. Moreover, the availability of e-books and digital publications further enriches their understanding of health-related matters and equips them with valuable insights to make informed choices.

By engaging in self-directed research and utilizing internet-based strategies, individuals can augment their understanding of various health conditions, treatments, and wellness practices. This empowers them to adopt proactive measures for preventive care and treatment, thereby enhancing their overall well-being. Additionally, the ease of access to diverse healthcare resources on the internet fosters a culture of continuous learning and self-improvement in managing personal health and wellness.

The integration of internet-based self-care practices not only benefits individuals but also presents opportunities for governments to streamline and enhance healthcare delivery. By promoting self-care through internet resources, governments can alleviate the burden on traditional healthcare systems, thereby optimizing resources and reducing strain on public healthcare facilities. This can lead to a more efficient allocation of healthcare resources and better management of healthcare demand, ultimately contributing to improved public health outcomes.

By facilitating and promoting self-care through internet resources, governments can cultivate a culture of health freedom and individual empowerment. Empowering individuals to be proactive in managing their health not only fosters a sense of personal responsibility but also contributes to a more resilient and informed society. Individuals who are well-informed and engaged in self-care are better positioned to take charge of their health, leading to improved overall health and well-being at the societal level.

Legal recognition and assurance of human freedom in healthcare are pivotal steps towards fostering a healthcare landscape that promotes individual autonomy, self-care, and informed decision-making. By leveraging internet resources, individuals can proactively engage in self-care, access valuable health information, and make informed choices for their well-being. This not only empowers individuals to take control of their health but also presents opportunities for governments to enhance public health outcomes and foster a culture of health freedom and individual empowerment.

There are key elements in the legal recognition and assurance of human freedom by governments which are paramount in preventing criminal activities surrounding the access and use of medicine. When governments grant legal recognition to human freedom, individuals are empowered to make their own health decisions, thereby reducing the reliance on healthcare centers and professionals. This freedom enables individuals to take charge of their health and well-being, allowing them to utilize their time effectively and become more self-reliant in managing their healthcare needs. The ability to become self-sufficient in health management not only empowers individuals but also reduces the potential for criminal activities in the healthcare sector.

When individuals take on the role of being their own doctors through the use of internet resources, they can access a wealth of information and research about their illnesses and potential treatments. This can lead to the formulation of effective strategies in managing their health using various online resources, such as e-books and reputable medical websites. Leveraging these online resources can enable individuals to make informed decisions about their healthcare, thereby reducing the reliance on traditional healthcare providers and facilities. This shift towards self-care and self-education can promote a more proactive approach to health management, ultimately leading to a healthier and more informed populace.

In contrast, the freedom to access medical information and resources online also presents opportunities for governments to create and implement simple and secure platforms that facilitate and promote health freedom. By leveraging the power of the internet and digital resources, governments can design user-friendly platforms that provide valuable health information and support to individuals, thereby fostering a culture of informed health decisions and self-care. This, in turn, can lead to a population that is more equipped to take charge of their health and well-being, ultimately reducing the burden on traditional healthcare systems and professionals.

By ensuring legal recognition and assurance of human freedom, governments can lay the foundation for a society that is empowered to take charge of their health and well-being. This shift towards self-reliance and proactive health management not only reduces the potential for criminal activity but also fosters a population that is equipped to make informed decisions about their health. Moreover, the utilization of online resources for health information and self-care can alleviate the strain on healthcare facilities and professionals, thereby enabling a more effective allocation of resources within the healthcare sector. Ultimately, the promotion of health freedom leads to a population that is more informed, empowered, and capable of leading healthier lives.

Ensuring human freedom in the context of legal recognition by governments holds paramount importance in mitigating medicine-based criminal activities and elevating individual agency in healthcare decision-making. When individuals have the legal freedom to seek healthcare from a variety of sources, outside the traditional healthcare centers, they are empowered to take control of their well-being. This autonomy allows for efficient utilization of time and resources, reducing the reliance on specialized medical professionals for every health concern. Emphasizing self-care and the ability to take on the role of a proactive patient not only promotes personal responsibility but also fosters a sense of empowerment and self-reliance in managing one's health.

Granting legal recognition to individual autonomy in healthcare choices also highlights the potential for individuals to become their own advocates and practitioners through the use of online resources. With access to a wealth of information and medical literature available on the internet, individuals have the opportunity to educate themselves about various health conditions and treatment options. Empowering individuals to conduct thorough research about their health concerns online enables them to develop informed strategies, choose suitable interventions, and engage in constructive conversations with healthcare professionals.

This paradigm shift towards self-driven healthcare not only enhances individuals' ability to make well-informed decisions but also has the potential to reduce the burden on traditional healthcare systems. By utilizing internet resources and e-books, individuals can augment their understanding of medical conditions, treatments, and preventative measures, leading to a more proactive approach to personal health management. This proactive engagement with health-related information can contribute to the prevention of illnesses and the early detection of health issues, ultimately promoting a population that is more in tune with their health and well-being.

From a governmental perspective, recognizing and facilitating individuals' freedom in healthcare choices can contribute to the formulation of streamlined and secure pathways for accessing healthcare information and services. Governments have the opportunity to establish regulations and guidelines that facilitate safe and effective utilization of online healthcare resources. By fostering an environment that encourages the responsible use of internet-based healthcare information, governments can promote a culture of health literacy and self-empowerment. Furthermore, this approach can bolster efforts to develop policies that prioritize health freedom, ultimately leading to a populace that is better equipped to make sound healthcare decisions.

In conclusion, the legal recognition of human freedom in healthcare by governments is pivotal in curbing medicine-based criminal activities and enabling individuals to take control of their health with confidence. This recognition promotes a culture of self-care and proactive health management, reducing the reliance on traditional healthcare models and fostering a greater sense of personal responsibility. Empowering individuals to leverage internet resources, e-books, and other online tools for healthcare research and decision-making not only enhances their ability to make well-informed choices but also contributes to the overall resilience of healthcare systems. Through collaborative efforts between individuals, government, and healthcare providers, the pursuit of health freedom can pave the way for a society that is more informed, engaged, and proactive in safeguarding its well-being.

Chapter Six: Empowering Health Literacy: Navigating the Digital Landscape for Accurate Diagnosis and Wellness

In the often overwhelming landscape of health information available on the internet, the importance of avoiding misdiagnosis cannot be overstated. As individuals take it upon themselves to research their illnesses online, they navigate through a myriad of resources that range from reputable medical websites to personal blogs and forums. This journey demands a careful and critical approach, emphasizing the significance of discerning accurate information from misinformation. Harnessing the power of the internet to educate oneself about health can indeed be empowering, but it also comes with significant risks if not approached with caution.

As individuals delve into the sea of online health resources, utilizing strategies that promote accuracy and reliability becomes paramount. Relying solely on internet searches for self-diagnosis can often lead to misunderstandings or misinterpretations of symptoms, potentially resulting in unnecessary anxiety or incorrect treatments. Instead, incorporating a variety of reputable sources, such as medical journals, authoritative websites, and e-books, can provide a more holistic understanding of one's condition. By cross-referencing information across multiple sources, individuals can validate the accuracy of their findings and make more informed decisions regarding their health.

Furthermore, the utilization of e-books on the internet adds another layer of depth to the wealth of health information available online. These digital resources offer in-depth insights into various medical conditions, treatment options, and preventive measures, allowing individuals to expand their knowledge beyond surface-level information. By engaging with e-books authored by reputable healthcare professionals, individuals can gain valuable perspectives and practical guidance that can supplement their online research.

In the broader context of public health, individuals' ability to access reliable health information through internet resources can also have implications for government policies and initiatives. Governments can leverage the digital landscape to disseminate accurate health information, promote preventive care measures, and raise awareness about common health issues. By fostering a culture of health literacy and informed decision-making through digital platforms, governments can empower their citizens to take charge of their well-being and lead healthier lives.

Moreover, the intersection of internet resources and government-led health initiatives can pave the way for the development of simple and accessible tools that cater to the diverse needs of the population. Creating user-friendly platforms that offer reliable health information, interactive tools for symptom assessment, and guidance on navigating the healthcare system can enhance individuals' ability to make informed choices about their health. By prioritizing user experience and ensuring the credibility of the information provided, governments can contribute to a society where health freedom is not just a concept but a tangible reality for all.

When researching illnesses online, it's vital to stress the significance of accuracy and reliability in the information obtained. There is an abundance of health-related content available on the internet, ranging from e-books to medical websites. However, the lack of quality control and expertise in some of these sources can lead to misinformation and potential misdiagnosis. Therefore, individuals must learn to discern credible sources from unreliable ones and exercise caution in interpreting and applying the information found online.

Utilizing internet resources for health research presents an opportunity for individuals to adopt the best strategies for their well-being. This includes accessing reputable e-books and articles that provide in-depth insights into various medical conditions, preventive measures, and treatment options. By leveraging these resources effectively, individuals can gain a better understanding of their health concerns, empowering them to make informed decisions and seek appropriate medical advice when necessary.

The utilization of internet resources in health research has broader implications, extending to governments and public health initiatives. Governments can harness the potential of online platforms to disseminate accurate and accessible health information to the public. By creating simple and safe pathways for individuals to access reliable health resources, governments can

contribute to fostering a society that prioritizes health literacy and proactive healthcare management.

In addition to individual health empowerment, robust internet resources can facilitate the development of community-based health initiatives. Through online platforms, individuals can connect with support groups, access reliable health education materials, and participate in wellness programs tailored to their specific needs. This interconnectedness and accessibility can significantly contribute to promoting health freedom and well-being within communities.

The availability of reputable e-books and online resources allows individuals to familiarize themselves with diverse perspectives on health and wellness. By exploring a wide range of expert opinions and evidence-based information, individuals can develop a comprehensive understanding of various health-related topics. This, in turn, enables them to make more informed decisions about their well-being and pursue lifestyle choices that align with their health goals.

Harnessing internet resources for health research can contribute to advancing preventive healthcare on a broader scale. By accessing reliable information on disease prevention, early detection, and healthy lifestyle practices, individuals can proactively safeguard their health and well-being. This proactive approach also has the potential to alleviate the burden on healthcare systems by reducing the incidence of preventable illnesses and promoting overall public health.

As individuals become more adept at utilizing internet resources for health research, they can actively engage in shaping healthcare policies and advocating for improved access to quality healthcare. By leveraging their knowledge and experiences, individuals can contribute to constructive dialogues about healthcare reform, accessibility, and the equitable distribution of medical resources. Ultimately, this collective effort can drive positive change in healthcare systems and policy-making processes.

The effective utilization of internet resources for health research holds profound implications for individuals, communities, and governments alike. By prioritizing accuracy and reliability in online health information, individuals can adopt informed strategies for managing their well-being. Simultaneously, governments can leverage internet platforms to establish accessible and safe channels for disseminating reliable health information, ultimately contributing to a society where health freedom is prioritized and upheld.

In the digital age, the internet has become a go-to source for information. When individuals turn to the internet to research their illnesses, it's crucial to approach this information with caution. Misdiagnosis based on unreliable internet sources can have serious consequences, leading to incorrect treatment plans and delayed proper medical care.

To avoid the pitfalls of misdiagnosis, individuals must learn to discern credible information from dubious sources on the internet. Striving for accuracy and reliability is paramount when using online resources for health-related information. This includes cross-referencing information from reputable websites, medical journals, and verified healthcare professionals to validate the information found online.

Utilizing the best strategies available on the internet, such as accessing e-books on health topics, can empower individuals to make informed decisions about their well-being. E-books can offer valuable insights, guidance, and tips on managing health conditions, promoting preventive care, and adopting healthy lifestyle practices.

By harnessing the wealth of information available online, individuals can take a proactive approach to their health and well-being. They can educate themselves about common health concerns, symptoms to watch for, and when to seek professional medical help. This self-empowerment through internet resources can lead to better health outcomes and a sense of control over one's health.

Governments play a pivotal role in ensuring that citizens have access to accurate and reliable health information online. By promoting trustworthy websites, creating educational campaigns, and supporting initiatives that prioritize health literacy, governments can help individuals navigate the vast landscape of internet resources safely.

Creating simple and secure pathways for individuals to access reliable health information online is vital for promoting health freedom. Governments can establish guidelines for internet health resources, develop user-friendly platforms, and invest in digital health initiatives to ensure that everyone can make informed decisions about their health.

By fostering a culture of digital health literacy, governments can empower individuals to make informed choices about their well-being. This can lead to a healthier population, reduced healthcare costs, and improved quality of life for all. Investing in accessible and user-friendly online health resources is a step towards creating a society where health freedom is a fundamental right.

Through collaboration with healthcare professionals, technology experts, and policymakers, governments can create a digital ecosystem that prioritizes accuracy, transparency, and user safety. This collaborative effort can ensure that individuals have the tools and resources they need to navigate the complexities of online health information effectively.

Avoiding misdiagnosis when researching illnesses online and utilizing internet resources wisely can lead to better health outcomes and a greater sense of empowerment. By leveraging e-books, reliable websites, and government-supported initiatives, individuals can take charge of their health journey and make informed decisions that promote a life full of health freedom.

By incorporating these practices into our healthcare systems and digital landscapes, we can create a future where individuals are equipped with the knowledge and resources needed to lead healthier, more fulfilling lives. Let's ensure that everyone has the opportunity to access safe, reliable, and empowering health information online for a brighter, healthier tomorrow.

Introducing the concept of health literacy and the role it plays in enabling individuals to discern between trustworthy and unreliable health information is essential. Exploring how enhanced health literacy and access to accurate internet resources can contribute to informed decision-making and proactive healthcare management will add depth to the chapter's content. Throughout all these discussions, emphasizing the importance of collaboration with healthcare professionals and incorporating online health information into a comprehensive care plan will guide readers towards a balanced and informed approach to utilizing internet resources for health-related purposes.

Shifting the focus to the role of governments in ensuring safe and reliable internet resources for health information, we can delve into the potential policy interventions and initiatives that governments can implement to support citizens in accessing accurate and trustworthy health data. Drawing parallels to existing public health campaigns and initiatives can offer insightful analogies, showcasing the potential impact of governmental support in promoting health freedom and empowering individuals to make informed decisions about their well-being.

Highlighting practical examples of how certain countries or regions have successfully implemented straightforward and secure methods for citizens to access reliable health information online can serve as inspiration for potential solutions and strategies that can be advocated for in various contexts. Sharing success stories and case studies of government-led initiatives or public-private partnerships in promoting health literacy and safe internet resources will further reinforce the positive impact of government involvement in this realm.

When navigating the vast landscape of health information available online, it is crucial to emphasize the importance of avoiding misdiagnosis. Individuals often turn to the internet to understand their symptoms or diagnoses, however, the abundance of information can sometimes lead to confusion and misinterpretation. It is essential for individuals to approach online health research with caution and skepticism, being mindful of the limitations and inaccuracies that may be present in some sources.

In the realm of online health resources, individuals have access to a wealth of information that can aid in understanding their health conditions and treatment options. By utilizing reliable internet sources and e-books, individuals can equip themselves with valuable knowledge to make informed decisions about their health. Reading e-books on the internet can provide in-depth knowledge on specific health topics, offering guidance on preventive measures, treatment options, and lifestyle modifications that can contribute to overall well-being.

The utilization of internet resources for health-related strategies can empower individuals to take an active role in managing their health. By arming themselves with accurate and up-to-date information, individuals can make better decisions regarding their well-being, leading to improved health outcomes and a higher quality of life. Online platforms offer a convenient and accessible way for individuals to educate themselves about various health conditions, enabling them to proactively address their health concerns.

Governments play a crucial role in facilitating the dissemination of reliable health information online. By promoting safe and trustworthy online resources, governments can ensure that individuals have access to accurate and evidence-based information to make informed decisions about their health. Establishing simple and secure ways for people to access reliable health information can significantly enhance public health literacy and contribute to a healthier population.

Creating a supportive environment for individuals to navigate online health resources can help prevent misdiagnosis and promote health freedom. Governments can implement policies and initiatives that prioritize the availability of credible health information online, ensuring that individuals have access to accurate and reliable resources for their health-related queries. By fostering a culture of health literacy and empowerment, governments can enable individuals to make informed choices about their health and well-being.

The avoidance of misdiagnosis when conducting online health research is paramount for individuals seeking to understand their health conditions and treatment options accurately. Leveraging internet resources, including e-books, can equip individuals with the knowledge and tools necessary to make informed decisions about their health. Additionally, government support in creating safe and accessible online platforms for health information can enhance public health literacy and promote a life full of health freedom for individuals. By emphasizing the importance of accurate and reliable health information online, individuals can take proactive steps towards managing their health effectively and leading a healthier lifestyle.

The journey of researching illnesses online can be a double-edged sword – while it empowers individuals with information and resources to take charge of their health, it also poses risks of misinformation and misdiagnosis. It is crucial for individuals to utilize reputable online resources and e-books to ensure accurate and reliable information when managing their health.

By fostering a culture of cautious and informed self-research, individuals can equip themselves with the best strategies for addressing their health concerns when leveraging internet resources. This approach not only promotes self-advocacy but also encourages proactive health management, leading to better health outcomes for individuals.

The role of governments in facilitating safe and simple ways for people to access accurate health information online cannot be overstated. By investing in public health initiatives that promote credible online health resources, governments can empower citizens to make informed decisions about their health and well-being.

Harnessing the power of technology and digital platforms, governments can create a supportive environment where individuals can navigate the vast landscape of health information online with confidence. This not only enhances health literacy but also contributes to a society where individuals are equipped to make sound health choices and live a life full of health freedom.

Ultimately, the collaborative effort between individuals, healthcare providers, and governments in promoting accurate health information online is key to reducing the risks of misdiagnosis and ensuring that individuals have access to reliable resources for managing their health. By prioritizing health education and information dissemination, we can create a collective environment that fosters wellness and empowers individuals to take control of their health journey.

Embracing the potential of internet resources and e-books as tools for health empowerment requires a deliberate approach towards discernment and critical thinking. Individuals must be vigilant in assessing the credibility of sources and seek guidance from healthcare professionals to validate the information obtained online.

Through continuous education and awareness campaigns, governments can play a pivotal role in guiding individuals towards reputable online resources that support their health goals. By promoting a culture of digital health literacy, governments can pave the way for a healthier and more informed society, where individuals are equipped with the knowledge and skills to navigate the online health landscape effectively.

As we navigate the evolving healthcare landscape and the increasing role of technology in health information dissemination, it is imperative that we prioritize accuracy, reliability, and safety when accessing online resources. By embracing the opportunities presented by digital platforms, individuals can harness the power of information to make informed decisions about their health and well-being.

In conclusion, the synergy between individuals, internet resources, and government initiatives holds the potential to revolutionize the way we approach health management in the digital age. By leveraging the vast array of online resources available, individuals can arm themselves with the knowledge and tools necessary to lead a life full of health freedom, while governments can provide the necessary infrastructure and support to ensure that this journey is safe and empowering for all.

Chapter Seven: Safeguarding Health: Navigating Risks and Empowering Choices Through Online Resources

By promoting the utilization of reputable online resources, such as e-books and reliable websites, individuals can develop a better understanding of their health conditions and the available treatment options. This not only empowers them to actively participate in their healthcare journey but also serves as a preventive measure against falling victim to criminal activities that may target individuals seeking traditional healthcare services.

In today's digital age, the internet has become a vast repository of health-related information. Governments have the opportunity to promote and support the availability of safe, accurate, and easily accessible online health resources. By doing so, they contribute to the creation of a health-conscious society, where individuals have the tools and knowledge to make informed decisions about their well-being. Moreover, the availability of reliable online health information serves as a protective measure, mitigating the risks associated with criminal intentions that may target unsuspecting individuals seeking medical care in person.

As individuals become more adept at utilizing internet resources for health research, they are better equipped to navigate the intricacies of healthcare, identify potential risks, and make informed decisions about their well-being. This shift towards internet-based health strategies can ultimately foster a sense of health freedom, allowing individuals to take control of their health outcomes and reduce the potential vulnerability to criminal activities in traditional healthcare settings.

The establishment of safe and easily accessible online health resources not only benefits individuals but also contributes to the overall enhancement of public health. Government support and advocacy for reliable online health information can significantly impact the well-being of the populace, paving the way for a healthier and more informed society. It ultimately plays a pivotal role in creating a health-conscious environment where individuals are empowered to lead lives full of health freedom and well-being.

In the seventh chapter of the book, a crucial discussion revolves around the risks associated with seeking medical care in person. It delves into the potential threats of encountering criminal activities within traditional healthcare settings, emphasizing the importance of awareness and vigilance in such scenarios. By addressing these risks head-on, the narrative highlights the significance of understanding how individuals can safeguard themselves while accessing healthcare services.

Exploring the realm of online resources for research on illnesses and health strategies is paramount in empowering individuals to make well-informed decisions regarding their healthcare. This chapter accentuates the transformative role that the internet can play in providing individuals with the necessary tools and knowledge to navigate their health journey effectively. By advocating for the utilization of reputable online platforms, such as e-books and reliable websites, the narrative underscores the value of digital information in promoting health literacy and preventive measures against potential criminal schemes.

In today's digital landscape, the internet has emerged as a repository of valuable health-related information. The chapter underscores the opportunity for governments to endorse safe, accurate, and easily accessible online health resources. By supporting the proliferation of reliable digital health content, authorities contribute to cultivating a health-conscious populace capable of making informed decisions about their well-being. This initiative not only bolsters individual empowerment but also acts as a shield against criminal activities that may target individuals within traditional healthcare settings.

A pivotal aspect highlighted in the narrative is the enhancement of health literacy through online research avenues. As individuals refine their skills in utilizing internet resources for health-related inquiries, they become adept at discerning potential risks, identifying suitable treatment options, and actively participating in their healthcare decisions. This paradigm shift towards embracing internet-based health strategies fosters a culture of health autonomy, enabling individuals to proactively manage their health outcomes and reduce susceptibility to criminal intentions in conventional healthcare environments.

The promotion of safe and accessible online health resources extends beyond individual benefits to augment public health on a broader scale. The chapter underscores the role of government advocacy in endorsing reliable digital health information to bolster the well-being of the population. By championing the dissemination of trustworthy online health content, authorities contribute to nurturing a society that prioritizes health consciousness and informed decision-making. This concerted effort fortifies a conducive environment where individuals are empowered to lead healthy lifestyles and mitigate vulnerabilities to criminal activities in healthcare settings.

Ultimately, the narrative posits that the establishment of reliable online health resources is instrumental in shaping a healthier and more well-informed society. The collaborative efforts of governments, healthcare institutions, and digital platforms in promoting safe digital health information pave the way for a populace equipped with the knowledge and tools to navigate their health journeys successfully. This collective endeavor plays a pivotal role in fostering a culture of health freedom, where individuals are empowered to proactively engage with their well-being, thereby curbing the risks associated with criminal activities in traditional healthcare realms.

In the seventh chapter of the book, the focus is on the risks associated with seeking medical care in person and the potential for encountering criminal activities. It discusses how utilizing internet resources for research on illnesses and health strategies can empower individuals and serve as a safeguard against targeted criminal plans in traditional healthcare settings. By promoting the use of reputable online resources like e-books and reliable websites, individuals can gain a better understanding of their health conditions and available treatment options, empowering them to actively participate in their healthcare journey and protect against falling victim to criminal activities targeting traditional healthcare services.

In today's digital age, the internet is a vast repository of health-related information. Governments have the opportunity to promote and support the availability of safe, accurate, and easily accessible online health resources. This can contribute to the creation of a health-conscious society, where individuals have the tools and knowledge to make informed decisions about their well-being, and serve as a protective measure against criminal intentions targeting individuals seeking medical care in person.

As individuals become more adept at utilizing internet resources for health research, they are better equipped to navigate the intricacies of healthcare, identify potential risks, and make informed decisions about their well-being. This shift towards internet-based health strategies can ultimately foster a sense of health freedom, allowing individuals to take control of their health outcomes and reduce vulnerability to criminal activities in traditional healthcare settings.

The establishment of safe and easily accessible online health resources not only benefits individuals but also contributes to the overall enhancement of public health. Government support and advocacy for reliable online health information can significantly impact the well-being of the populace, paving the way for a healthier and more informed society. It ultimately plays a pivotal role in creating a health-conscious environment where individuals are empowered to lead lives full of health freedom and well-being.

In the seventh chapter of the book, the discussion of risks associated with seeking in-person medical care and potential criminal activities is paramount. This section emphasizes the importance of utilizing internet resources to conduct research on illnesses and health strategies, empowering individuals to make informed decisions about their health while safeguarding against criminal intent in traditional healthcare settings.

Promoting the use of reputable online resources, such as e-books and reliable websites, allows individuals to gain a better understanding of their health conditions and treatment options. This empowerment not only encourages active participation in one's healthcare journey but also serves as a preventive measure against falling victim to criminal activities targeting those seeking traditional healthcare services.

The seventh chapter of the book emphasizes the importance of addressing the risks associated with seeking medical care in person, especially concerning potential criminal activities individuals may encounter. The discussion highlights how conducting research on illnesses and health strategies using internet resources can empower individuals to make informed decisions about their health and serve as a safeguard against targeted criminal plans in traditional healthcare settings. This approach emphasizes promoting the utilization of reputable online resources, such as e-books and reliable websites, to develop a better understanding of health conditions and treatment options. This empowerment not only allows individuals to actively participate in their healthcare journey but also serves as a preventive measure against falling victim to criminal activities targeting those seeking traditional healthcare services.

In today's digital age, the internet has become a vast repository of health-related information, offering governments the opportunity to promote and support the availability of safe, accurate, and easily accessible online health resources. By doing so, they contribute to the creation of a health-conscious society, where individuals have the tools and knowledge to make informed decisions about their well-being. Moreover, the availability of reliable online health information serves as a protective measure, mitigating the risks associated with criminal intentions targeting unsuspecting individuals seeking medical care in person.

As individuals become more adept at utilizing internet resources for health research, they are better equipped to navigate the intricacies of healthcare, identify potential risks, and make informed decisions about their well-being. This shift towards internet-based health strategies can ultimately foster a sense of health freedom, allowing individuals to take control of their health outcomes and reduce vulnerability to criminal activities in traditional healthcare settings.

The establishment of safe and easily accessible online health resources not only benefits individuals but also contributes to the overall enhancement of public health. Government support and advocacy for reliable online health information can significantly impact the well-being of the populace, paving the way for a healthier and more informed society. It plays a pivotal role in creating a health-conscious environment where individuals are empowered to lead lives full of health freedom and well-being. This encourages individuals to become proactive in managing their health and promotes a sense of personal responsibility, ultimately contributing to improved overall health outcomes for society.

The seventh chapter of the book sheds light on the critical risks associated with seeking medical care in person, particularly in the context of potential criminal activities individuals may encounter. By delving into how research on illnesses and health strategies can be effectively conducted through internet resources, the chapter underscores the importance of empowering individuals to make informed decisions about their health while safeguarding against targeted criminal activities within traditional healthcare settings.

By advocating for the utilization of reputable online resources like e-books and reliable websites, individuals are encouraged to enhance their understanding of health conditions and available treatment options. This not only empowers them to actively engage in their healthcare journey but also serves as a protective measure against becoming victims of criminal schemes that often target individuals seeking conventional healthcare services.

The seventh chapter of the book sheds light on the critical risks associated with seeking medical care in person, particularly in the context of potential criminal activities individuals may encounter. By delving into how research on illnesses and health strategies can be effectively conducted through internet resources, the chapter underscores the importance of empowering individuals to make informed decisions about their health while safeguarding against targeted criminal activities within traditional healthcare settings.

By advocating for the utilization of reputable online resources like e-books and reliable websites, individuals are encouraged to enhance their understanding of health conditions and available treatment options. This not only empowers them to actively engage in their healthcare journey but also serves as a protective measure against becoming victims of criminal schemes that often target individuals seeking conventional healthcare services.

The discussion in the seventh chapter underscores the importance of leveraging internet resources to address the risks associated with seeking medical care and potential criminal activities. This approach not only empowers individuals to make informed decisions about their health but also serves as a safeguard against targeted criminal plans encountered in traditional healthcare settings.

By promoting reputable online resources, individuals can develop a better understanding of their health conditions and treatment options, empowering them to actively participate in their healthcare journey and serving as a preventive measure against falling victim to criminal activities in traditional healthcare services.

The discussion on the risks associated with seeking medical care in person, particularly in the context of potential criminal activities, underscores the paramount importance of utilizing internet resources for health research. By emphasizing the empowerment and security that online health information can provide, individuals are urged to take charge of their well-being with informed decisions.

The exploration of utilizing reliable online resources such as e-books and verified websites unveils a proactive approach to understanding health conditions and treatment options. This strategy not only fosters active patient engagement but also acts as a shield against malicious intents targeting those seeking traditional healthcare services.

As we navigate the digital landscape of health information, governments are presented with the opportunity to endorse and ensure the availability of trustworthy online health resources. By facilitating access to accurate and understandable health data, authorities contribute to a society where informed choices drive well-being and act as a barrier to potential criminal activities in healthcare settings.

The increasing proficiency in harnessing internet resources for health research equips individuals with the skills to assess healthcare intricacies, recognize risks, and secure their well-being through knowledgeable decisions. This shift towards internet-driven health strategies cultivates a realm of health empowerment, enabling individuals to steer their health trajectories and diminish susceptibility to criminal activities within traditional healthcare realms.

Reflecting on the implications of harnessing internet-based health approaches, individuals are encouraged to embrace a sense of health freedom, where autonomy over health outcomes is fostered. This empowerment not only redresses the power dynamics in healthcare but also fortifies defenses against criminal undertakings, emphasizing the importance of informed choices in safeguarding one's health journey.

The establishment of secure and accessible online health repositories presents an avenue for collective advancement in public health agendas. Through governmental support and advocacy for reliable health information online, the societal landscape shifts towards a health-conscious environment, steering individuals towards a path of self-empowerment and informed decision-making.

By delving into the realm of online health resources, individuals are equipped to discern credible sources, gain knowledge, and thwart potential threats in healthcare scenarios. The evolving landscape of internet-driven health strategies paves the way for a future where individuals are active participants in their health management, reducing susceptibility to criminal activities through strategic decision-making.

The synergy between understanding the risks of traditional healthcare encounters and leveraging internet resources for health research underscores the pivotal role of education and accessibility in shaping health outcomes. Empowering individuals with the tools to navigate online health information not only enhances personal well-being but also fortifies defenses against malicious activities targeting vulnerable populations seeking healthcare services.

The narrative on mitigating risks associated with seeking medical care by advocating for internet-based health research advocates for a shift towards health empowerment and informed decision-making. By fostering a culture of health literacy and supporting reliable online resources, individuals and authorities alike contribute to a healthier, more secure society where knowledge acts as a shield against potential harm in traditional healthcare settings.

In the seventh chapter of the book, the focus is on the risks associated with seeking medical care in person and the potential criminal activities individuals may encounter. Not only does the chapter emphasize the importance of utilizing internet resources for health research to empower individuals to make informed decisions about their health, but it also highlights how it can serve as a safeguard against targeted criminal plans that may be encountered in traditional healthcare settings.

By promoting the use of reputable online resources such as e-books and reliable websites, the chapter underscores how individuals can develop a better understanding of their health conditions and available treatment options. This proactive approach not only empowers individuals to actively participate in their healthcare journey but also serves as a preventive measure against falling victim to criminal activities targeting individuals seeking traditional healthcare services.

In today's digital age, the internet has become a vast repository of health-related information, and the chapter emphasizes the opportunity for governments to promote and support the availability of safe, accurate, and easily accessible online health resources. By doing so, they contribute to the creation of a health-conscious society where individuals have the tools and knowledge to make informed decisions about their well-being. Additionally, the availability of reliable online health information serves as a protective measure, mitigating the risks associated with criminal intentions targeting unsuspecting individuals seeking medical care in person.

As individuals become more adept at using internet resources for health research, they are better equipped to navigate the intricacies of healthcare, identify potential risks, and make informed decisions about their well-being. This shift towards internet-based health strategies can ultimately foster a sense of health freedom, allowing individuals to take control of their health outcomes and reduce potential vulnerability to criminal activities in traditional healthcare settings.

The establishment of safe and easily accessible online health resources not only benefits individuals but also contributes to the overall enhancement of public health. The chapter emphasizes that government support and advocacy for reliable online health information can significantly impact the well-being of the populace, paving the way for a healthier and more informed society. It ultimately plays a pivotal role in creating a health-conscious environment where individuals are empowered to lead lives full of health freedom and well-being.

Chapter Eight: Empowering Health Literacy: Navigating Knowledge in the Digital Age

The accessibility of e-books and other online resources offers individuals the opportunity to expand their knowledge base on a diverse range of health-related topics. Whether it's understanding specific illnesses, exploring preventative strategies, or delving into treatment options, the wealth of information available online contributes to the development of well-informed and proactive individuals. Through self-education and research, individuals can gain a deeper insight into their health, demystifying complex medical concepts, and fostering a sense of confidence in managing their well-being.

The bond between individuals and the knowledge amassed through online resources plays a pivotal role in shaping them into authentic advocates for their health. By actively engaging with e-books and other online platforms, individuals can cultivate a sense of responsibility towards their own well-being, transcending passive reliance on external healthcare authorities. This proactive approach not only fosters a genuine understanding of health-related matters but also instills a sense of empowerment, positioning individuals as active participants in their healthcare journey.

The significance of individuals taking charge of their health through self-education extends beyond personal empowerment, resonating with broader implications for public health and governance. As individuals become more adept at leveraging online resources for self-education, they contribute to the cultivation of a society that values health freedom and informed decision-making. This shift towards self-empowerment serves as a catalyst for prompting governments to devise simpler and safer avenues for individuals to access credible health information, thereby fostering a society where health literacy and autonomy are foundational principles.

Recognizing the transformative potential of individuals embracing the role of self-educated advocates for their health, it becomes evident that nurturing this bond with knowledge through e-books and online resources is instrumental in fortifying a collective commitment to well-being. By championing the cultivation of genuine doctors for oneself, societies can pave the way for a paradigm shift in healthcare culture, where individuals are empowered to make conscientious choices and actively contribute to the creation of a healthier community. Therefore, the strengthening of the bond between people and knowledge available online not only serves to benefit individual health outcomes but also holds the promise of revitalizing public health dynamics on a larger scale.

In the eighth chapter of my book, it's imperative to emphasize the profound significance of strengthening the bond between individuals and the knowledge they can acquire through reading e-books and utilizing various online resources. This chapter serves as an opportunity to delve into how empowering individuals to become genuine doctors for themselves, through access to credible online information, can fundamentally transform their approach to health and well-being. By advocating for the utilization of e-books and diverse online resources, this chapter will highlight the pivotal role of knowledge empowerment in fostering a proactive and informed healthcare approach.

Encouraging the utilization of e-books and diverse online resources is essential in empowering individuals to take charge of their health journey. Providing access to a wealth of information through these channels enables people to expand their understanding of various health conditions, treatment options, and preventive measures. This, in turn, cultivates a sense of ownership and responsibility for one's well-being, thereby contributing to the formation of a genuine partnership between individuals and their health.

Advocating for the usage of e-books and other online resources lays the groundwork for individuals to become their own genuine doctors. Access to these resources equips individuals with the necessary tools to make informed decisions about their health, promoting a proactive and preventive approach to wellness. By fostering a culture of self-education and empowerment, individuals can adopt a more comprehensive understanding of their health needs and actively engage in promoting their overall well-being.

Importantly, the utilization of e-books and various online resources not only empowers individuals but also presents an opportunity for governments to create straightforward and secure pathways for people to live lives filled with health freedom. By promoting and supporting the

availability of safe, accurate, and easily accessible online health resources, governments can contribute to the creation of a society where individuals have the means to make informed decisions about their health and well-being.

This emphasis on e-books and online resources as tools for becoming genuine doctors for oneself plays a crucial role in promoting health literacy and fostering a sense of empowerment among individuals. Through access to diverse digital resources, individuals can broaden their knowledge base, enabling them to navigate the complexities of healthcare with confidence and understanding. This proactive engagement with health-related information can lead to a heightened sense of agency and personal responsibility, ultimately contributing to the development of a society characterized by health-conscious and well-informed individuals.

Additionally, promoting the utilization of e-books and other online resources in healthcare underscores the transformative potential of digital platforms in advancing public health. By actively encouraging individuals to seek knowledge and information from online sources, governments and health authorities can effectively amplify the dissemination of crucial health-related insights. This proactive dissemination of information serves to elevate public awareness and understanding of prevailing health challenges, thereby bolstering the overall health literacy of the populace.

Emphasizing the importance of strengthening the bond between individuals and their health knowledge through accessible online resources aligns with the evolving landscape of healthcare in the digital era. By fostering a culture of continuous learning and self-empowerment, individuals can proactively engage with diverse health-related materials, thereby fostering a sense of personal agency in managing their well-being. This fundamental shift towards knowledge empowerment redefines the traditional patient-doctor dynamic, encouraging individuals to assume an active role in their own health maintenance and decision-making processes.

The elevation of e-books and other online resources as vehicles for promoting health consciousness and freedom represents a significant step towards fostering a society where individuals are equipped with the necessary tools to make informed decisions about their well-being. This deliberate emphasis on knowledge acquisition through digital channels nurtures a culture of responsibility and self-reliance, ultimately contributing to the cultivation of a community where individuals are empowered to lead lives characterized by health freedom and informed decision-making.

Advocating for the utilization of e-books and various online resources underscores the transformative potential of digital platforms in reshaping traditional healthcare paradigms. By championing the adoption of digital resources as proponents of health empowerment, individuals can harness the vast repository of health-related information available online, ultimately cultivating a proactive and informed approach to wellness. This shift towards digital literacy not only serves to enhance individual knowledge but also contributes to the collective advancement of public health initiatives, thereby fostering a society characterized by greater health consciousness and self-advocacy.

Promoting the utilization of e-books and diverse online resources as catalysts for becoming genuine doctors for oneself represents a multidimensional approach to healthcare advocacy. By actively supporting the utilization of digital platforms as vehicles for knowledge acquisition and self-empowerment, individuals can transcend traditional healthcare limitations, thereby nurturing a community marked by individual agency and proactive engagement with health-related information. This concerted effort towards fostering a society of informed and empowered individuals contributes to the creation of a health-conscious environment, ultimately paving the way for individuals to lead lives abundant with health freedom and well-being.

In the eighth chapter of my book, it is pivotal to delve into the significance of strengthening the bond between individuals and the knowledge they can acquire through reading e-books and utilizing various online resources. This chapter focuses on the journey of becoming a genuine doctor for oneself, emphasizing the role of accessible information in promoting health literacy and individual empowerment.

The availability of e-books and online resources plays a fundamental role in shaping individuals into their own health advocates. By engaging with diverse sources of information, individuals can expand their knowledge base and develop a deeper understanding of health-related matters. This, in turn, equips them with the tools to proactively manage their well-being and make informed decisions about their health.

It is vital to emphasize that embracing the wealth of knowledge available through e-books and online platforms can significantly contribute to laying the groundwork for individuals to become more self-reliant in managing their health. By fostering a strong connection between people and accessible knowledge, the foundation is laid for a shift towards a proactive approach to healthcare, empowering individuals to take charge of their well-being and make informed decisions.

Exploring the depths of online resources can aid in nurturing a sense of responsibility and ownership over one's health. The act of engaging with a diverse range of health-related materials promotes critical thinking and encourages individuals to question, analyze, and synthesize information, thereby fostering a deeper understanding of health-related concepts and strategies.

As individuals embark on their journey to become genuine doctors for themselves, the role of accessible online resources cannot be overstated. These platforms not only provide a treasure trove of health-related information but also contribute to the cultivation of a health-conscious mindset. By promoting a culture of continuous learning and self-education, individuals are empowered to embrace a proactive stance towards their health, ultimately leading to a heightened sense of health freedom and autonomy.

Additionally, the utilization of e-books and online resources serves as a catalyst for the development of a symbiotic relationship between individuals and their health. Access to reliable and comprehensive information fosters a sense of empowerment, enabling individuals to navigate the complexities of healthcare with confidence and assertiveness. This, in turn, strengthens the connection between people and the knowledge essential for making well-informed decisions about their health.

The establishment of a strong bond between individuals and accessible knowledge paves the way for the creation of simple and safe pathways for people to lead lives replete with health freedom. By harnessing the potential of e-books and online resources, governments have the opportunity to facilitate the dissemination of essential health information to the populace, thereby promoting a culture of informed decision-making and proactive health management.

It is crucial to recognize that nurturing the bond between individuals and the abundance of knowledge available online can also serve as a catalyst for broader societal changes. As individuals become adept at leveraging online resources for their health-related inquiries, it sets the stage for a collective shift towards a more health-conscious society, driven by informed choices and a proactive approach to well-being.

The embrace of e-books and online platforms as sources of health-related information transcends individual benefits and extends to the realm of public health. By nurturing a culture of self-education and informed decision-making, the populace becomes better equipped to contribute to a healthier and more resilient society, where individuals are adept at safeguarding their own well-being and that of their communities.

The availability of e-books and online resources plays a fundamental role in shaping individuals into their own health advocates. By engaging with diverse sources of information, individuals can expand their knowledge base and develop a deeper understanding of health-related matters. This, in turn, equips them with the tools to proactively manage their well-being and make informed decisions about their health.

It is vital to emphasize that embracing the wealth of knowledge available through e-books and online platforms can significantly contribute to laying the groundwork for individuals to become more self-reliant in managing their health. By fostering a strong connection between people and accessible knowledge, the foundation is laid for a shift towards a proactive approach to healthcare, empowering individuals to take charge of their well-being and make informed decisions.

Exploring the depths of online resources can aid in nurturing a sense of responsibility and ownership over one's health. The act of engaging with a diverse range of health-related materials promotes critical thinking and encourages individuals to question, analyze, and synthesize information, thereby fostering a deeper understanding of health-related concepts and strategies.

As individuals embark on their journey to become genuine doctors for themselves, the role of accessible online resources cannot be overstated. These platforms not only provide a treasure trove of health-related information but also contribute to the cultivation of a health-conscious mindset. By promoting a culture of continuous learning and self-education, individuals are empowered to embrace a proactive stance towards their health, ultimately leading to a heightened sense of health freedom and autonomy.

Additionally, the utilization of e-books and online resources serves as a catalyst for the development of a symbiotic relationship between individuals and their health. Access to reliable and comprehensive information fosters a sense of empowerment, enabling individuals to navigate the complexities of healthcare with confidence and assertiveness. This, in turn, strengthens the connection between people and the knowledge essential for making well-informed decisions about their health.

The establishment of a strong bond between individuals and accessible knowledge paves the way for the creation of simple and safe pathways for people to lead lives replete with health freedom. By harnessing the potential of e-books and online resources, governments have the opportunity to facilitate the dissemination of essential health information to the populace, thereby promoting a culture of informed decision-making and proactive health management.

It is crucial to recognize that nurturing the bond between individuals and the abundance of knowledge available online can also serve as a catalyst for broader societal changes. As individuals become adept at leveraging online resources for their health-related inquiries, it sets the stage for a collective shift towards a more health-conscious society, driven by informed choices and a proactive approach to well-being.

The embrace of e-books and online platforms as sources of health-related information transcends individual benefits and extends to the realm of public health. By nurturing a culture of self-education and informed decision-making, the populace becomes better equipped to contribute to a healthier and more resilient society, where individuals are adept at safeguarding their own well-being and that of their communities.

The eighth chapter of my book serves as a profound exploration of the transformative power of strengthening the connection between individuals and the wealth of knowledge available through e-books and online resources. This emphasis on fostering a sense of agency and responsibility in managing personal health not only empowers individuals but also paves the way for societal changes that promote health freedom and well-being.

Strengthening the bond between individuals and the knowledge they can attain through various resources, including e-books and online platforms, is crucial in the journey towards becoming a genuine doctor of oneself. By exploring the vast array of reading materials available online, individuals can enhance their understanding of various subjects, including healthcare practices and principles. This access to knowledge empowers individuals to take charge of their well-being and make informed decisions regarding their health. As the global landscape of information continues to evolve, leveraging e-books and online resources becomes essential for individuals aspiring to become well-rounded and knowledgeable individuals in the medical field.

The significance of fostering a strong connection between people and the wealth of knowledge offered by e-books and online resources cannot be overstated. By actively engaging with credible sources online, individuals can expand their horizons and deepen their understanding of essential medical concepts. This, in turn, equips them with the necessary tools to navigate the complex realm of healthcare with confidence and expertise. Moreover, the seamless access to information available online facilitates continuous learning and self-improvement, thereby enabling individuals to cultivate their skills and expertise effectively.

In addition to benefiting individuals on a personal level, strengthening the bond between people and the knowledge available online holds immense potential for governmental initiatives aimed at promoting public health and well-being. Through strategic collaborations and partnerships with online platforms, governments can develop streamlined and secure avenues for individuals to access vital health information. Such initiatives not only empower individuals to make informed choices regarding their health but also contribute to the creation of a society that prioritizes wellness and preventative care. By embracing e-books and online resources, governments can pave the way for citizens to lead healthy, fulfilling lives.

Emphasizing the importance of leveraging e-books and online resources in the pursuit of becoming a genuine doctor of oneself underscores the transformative power of continuous learning and self-discovery. In today's digital age, the abundance of information available online allows individuals to delve into diverse sources of knowledge and gain valuable insights into various aspects of medicine and healthcare. By immersing themselves in relevant literature and resources, individuals can cultivate a holistic understanding of health-related topics and enhance their ability to make well-informed decisions about their well-being.

Recognizing the pivotal role of online platforms in strengthening the bond between knowledge and individuals underscores the evolution of healthcare practices in the digital era. The accessibility of e-books and online resources enables aspiring medical professionals to stay abreast of the latest advancements and developments in the field, thereby sharpening their skills and competencies. This continuous engagement with educational materials fosters a culture of lifelong learning and professional growth, positioning individuals as proactive agents of change in the healthcare landscape. By embracing digital resources, individuals can embark on a transformative journey towards becoming genuine doctors of themselves.

In the context of government initiatives aimed at promoting health freedom and well-being, the synergy between individuals and online knowledge resources emerges as a potent force for societal progress. By harnessing the power of e-books and online platforms, governments can empower citizens to take charge of their health and wellness, thereby fostering a culture of self-care and prevention. The widespread availability of online resources not only enhances individuals' access to critical health information but also serves as a catalyst for collective action towards building healthier communities. Through collaborative efforts with online publishers, governments can establish inclusive and user-friendly platforms that provide citizens with the tools they need to lead fulfilling and healthy lives.

The transformative potential of strengthening the bond between individuals and online knowledge resources extends beyond personal growth to encompass broader societal benefits. By encouraging individuals to engage with e-books and online platforms in their pursuit of medical knowledge, governments can foster a culture of innovation and collaboration within the healthcare sector. This shared commitment to continuous learning and knowledge-sharing lays the foundation for a more inclusive and resilient healthcare system, wherein individuals are empowered to make well-informed decisions about their health and well-being. The convergence of digital resources and individual agency paves the way for a future where informed citizens play an active role in shaping the healthcare landscape.

Emphasizing the importance of integrating e-books and online resources into individuals' quest to become genuine doctors of themselves underscores the transformative impact of digital literacy on health outcomes. In an age where information is readily accessible at the click of a button, individuals have the unprecedented opportunity to deepen their understanding of health-related topics and empower themselves to make informed choices. By leveraging e-books and online platforms, individuals can transcend traditional boundaries of learning and explore a wealth of knowledge that enriches their personal and professional lives. This digital revolution in education and self-discovery heralds a new era in which individuals are equipped with the tools they need to navigate the complexities of modern healthcare with confidence and efficacy.

By advocating for the integration of e-books and online resources into everyday learning practices, individuals can harness the collective wisdom of the digital world to advance their personal growth and development. The democratization of knowledge through online platforms opens doors to new opportunities for individuals to explore diverse perspectives and insights on healthcare and wellness.

Chapter 9: Embracing Knowledge for Personal Empowerment

As the journey through the preceding chapters has illuminated, the transformative potential of embracing a deeper connection to knowledge, particularly through e-books and online resources, is resoundingly clear. Building upon the foundation laid in the previous chapter, Chapter 9 delves further into the overarching theme of empowerment through knowledge acquisition and application. This chapter seeks to elucidate the profound impact of knowledge on personal agency, particularly in the realm of health and well-being.

In a world inundated with a wealth of digital information, the cultivation of robust decision-making skills in managing personal health has never been more crucial. Chapter 9 takes a strategic approach in unraveling the layers of agency and responsibility that individuals can harness when equipped with the tools to navigate through the vast expanse of online knowledge. Furthermore, the message resonating through this chapter transcends individual impact, stretching into the societal fabric and highlighting the potential for broader systemic changes that foster health freedom and overall well-being for communities at large.

Articulating the intersection between education, digital literacy, and health, the ninth chapter embarks on a thought-provoking exploration of how the harnessing of online resources can serve as a catalyst for individual empowerment. By dissecting real-world examples and case studies, this chapter aims to make tangible the intangible concept of digital empowerment and the pivotal role it plays in shaping a healthier and more informed society.

This chapter endeavors to push past the traditional boundaries of information consumption, emphasizing the proactive role individuals can embody in curating, evaluating, and applying knowledge in ways that directly influence their health landscape. By embracing the digital evolution in information acquisition, individuals can elevate their levels of self-advocacy and take ownership of their well-being, thereby reshaping the dynamics of healthcare decision-making and resource utilization.

Through an amalgamation of research-backed insights, personal anecdotes, and expert perspectives, Chapter 9 seeks to cohesively weave a narrative that underscores the bridge between individual knowledge empowerment and the overarching collective benefits that can be reaped from a populace well-versed in navigating the digital sphere for health-related guidance.

This chapter is not confined to a mere philosophical exposition on the intrinsic value of digital literacy and health agency; rather, it aims to be a practical roadmap for readers to navigate the intricate landscape of e-books and online resources, distilling actionable strategies for cultivating a well-informed and empowered approach to managing personal health.

As the sequential progression of this book unfolds, Chapter 9 emerges as a linchpin in elucidating the pivotal role of knowledge as a vehicle for personal empowerment, advocating for a seismic shift in the way individuals engage with and leverage digital resources for their holistic well-being.

In essence, the ninth chapter serves as a testament to the potency of knowledge as the catalyst for individual and communal transformation, positioning digital literacy as the cornerstone of a paradigm shift towards health empowerment and liberation.

As the narrative of this chapter unfolds, it becomes abundantly clear that the reliable availability of emergency health services is not merely a convenience but a vital necessity for individuals facing health crises. Understanding the pivotal role of emergency health services as a lifeline for those unable to independently address their medical needs, this chapter staunchly advocates for the comprehensive and secure provision of such services by governments and healthcare systems. The need for prompt and effective emergency care is especially resonant for individuals grappling with serious health conditions, where the ability to self-diagnose or self-manage becomes untenable, reinforcing the indispensability of accessible and reliable emergency healthcare.

It is imperative to recognize that individuals facing a significant deterioration in their health are often incapacitated to the extent that the capacity to independently "become the doctor" to themselves is a far-reaching aspiration. In such circumstances, the role of emergency health services in swiftly and competently addressing emergent medical needs becomes not just desirable, but an absolute imperative. This chapter underscores the criticality of governments in ensuring the secure and unfettered access to emergency healthcare, emphasizing the moral and ethical obligations incumbent upon healthcare systems to readily serve individuals during their most vulnerable moments without compromise.

The interplay between an individual's deteriorating health and their ability to actively engage in self-care cannot be overstated. In the face of debilitating health constraints, the reliance on emergency health services as the bastion of immediate and specialized care stands as a non-negotiable imperative. This chapter staunchly advocates for the fortification of emergency healthcare infrastructure and resources, reiterating the irrefutable rights of individuals to access swiftly deployed medical interventions during crises, irrespective of their socio-economic standing or geographic location.

The chapter accentuates the reciprocal benefits of bolstering emergency health services as an investment in societal resilience and well-being. By safeguarding individuals from the adverse consequences of delayed or inaccessible emergency care, governments and healthcare agencies play a pivotal role in fostering a more resilient and empowered populace. The inseparable connection between accessible emergency health services and the mitigation of preventable health complications underlies the foundational premises expounded in this chapter, compelling stakeholders to recognize the broader ramifications of fortifying emergency healthcare as a buffer against avoidable suffering and adverse health outcomes.

Emphasizing the indispensable obligation of governments to uphold the sanctity of life and ensure the unfailing provision of emergency healthcare services, this chapter underscores the ethical mandate for robust emergency care infrastructure. The inextricable link between the effective administration of emergency healthcare and the preservation of human dignity steers the discourse towards a resounding call for governments to prioritize and fortify emergency health services. The moral imperative of championing the accessibility and reliability of emergency healthcare regardless of an individual's circumstances or background looms large as the foundational ethos driving this impassioned plea for holistic and secure emergency care provision.

In recognizing the irreplaceable role of emergency health services as the indispensable safety net for vulnerable individuals in crisis, this chapter fervently advocates for the formulation and implementation of robust policies that ensure the secure and equitable availability of emergency care. The ensuing discourse traverses beyond theoretical postulations, steering towards a practical outline of the fundamental principles that must underpin the governance and administration of emergency health services. Stressing the exigent need for proactive investment in emergency healthcare infrastructure, the narrative pivots towards a strategic blueprint for governments and healthcare systems to effectuate the reliable and secure delivery of life-saving interventions to those in need.

The implications of inadequate or unsecured emergency healthcare provision reverberate far beyond the immediate purview of individual health crises, signifying a systemic vulnerability that permeates the fabric of societal well-being. This chapter underscores the interdependence of a secure emergency health system with broader public health outcomes, elucidating the profound ramifications of unattended emergent health needs on the overall health landscape. By elevating the discourse beyond the individualistic lens and dissecting the systemic reverberations of compromised emergency healthcare, the chapter palpably illustrates the intrinsic interconnectedness of robust emergency care infrastructure with communal health resilience.

The ninth chapter amplifies the clarion call for governments to meticulously and ardently fortify emergency health services, recognizing it as a sine qua non for individual and communal well-being. The impassioned plea articulated in this chapter is underscored by a fervent advocacy for the realization of universal and secure emergency healthcare as an inviolable prerogative for all individuals, emblematic of a society's collective commitment to safeguarding the sanctity of life and promoting health equity.

In Chapter 9 of my book, the focus shifts towards a crucial aspect of healthcare - the provision of secure and reliable emergency health services by governments as a fundamental necessity for public well-being. It delves deep into the intrinsic value of emergency health services, emphasizing that individuals often need prompt medical assistance when they are in a state of health crisis where they are unable to address their own medical needs effectively.

The chapter elaborates on the critical role that governments play in ensuring that emergency health services are not just available but also secure and accessible to all individuals. It underscores the importance of a robust emergency healthcare system that is well-equipped to respond swiftly to people's urgent medical needs, especially during times of dire health emergencies. This reliability and accessibility of emergency services are essential in safeguarding the welfare and health outcomes of individuals in communities.

By advocating for the establishment of secure emergency health services, the chapter highlights the significance of governments prioritizing the allocation of resources, infrastructure, and trained personnel to effectively manage and operate emergency healthcare facilities. This strategic investment serves as a safeguard against situations where individuals may find themselves incapacitated due to health crises and urgently require professional medical intervention.

The narrative in Chapter 9 acknowledges the reality that individuals cannot be expected to solely rely on self-treatment or self-diagnosis when faced with severe health conditions that render them incapable of taking on the role of a healthcare provider to themselves. In such challenging circumstances, the availability of reliable emergency health services becomes a lifeline for individuals, ensuring timely access to critical medical care that can potentially save lives and alleviate suffering.

The chapter emphasizes that governments bear a significant responsibility in creating a healthcare ecosystem where emergency services are not only accessible but also instill a sense of security and trust among the population. This sense of security is paramount in encouraging individuals to seek medical assistance promptly when faced with health emergencies, rather than hesitating due to concerns about the reliability or availability of emergency healthcare services.

Moreover, Chapter 9 elucidates on the interconnectedness between the efficiency of emergency health services and the overall public health outcomes within a society. Secure and dependable emergency healthcare facilities not only address individual health crises but also contribute to the broader goal of enhancing community health resilience, reducing morbidity, and promoting timely interventions that can mitigate the spread of infectious diseases or other health threats.

Within the discourse of emergency health services, the chapter raises important questions regarding the adequacy of emergency response protocols, the training of emergency medical personnel, and the strategic coordination between healthcare providers, emergency responders, and government agencies. These considerations are pivotal in ensuring that emergency health services operate seamlessly to address the diverse medical needs of individuals across different health emergencies.

Additionally, the narrative expounded in Chapter 9 underscores the imperative for governments to engage in proactive measures aimed at fortifying emergency health services through continuous evaluation, improvement, and adaptation to evolving healthcare challenges. This proactive approach involves investing in cutting-edge technologies, enhancing emergency preparedness strategies, and fostering collaborations with other healthcare stakeholders to strengthen the resilience of emergency healthcare systems.

Ultimately, the essence of Chapter 9 lies in advocating for a comprehensive and resilient emergency healthcare framework that not only addresses the immediate medical needs of individuals in crisis but also reflects a broader societal commitment to prioritizing the health and well-being of all citizens. By emphasizing the significance of secure and accessible emergency health services, the chapter champions a healthcare ethos that recognizes the indispensable role of governments in safeguarding public health through robust emergency medical interventions.

Crafting an influential and engaging introductory paragraph to the 9th chapter of my book requires attention to detail and a thorough understanding of the importance of emergency health services in society. By delving into the profound responsibility that governments carry in ensuring the security and reliability of emergency health services, the narrative can underscore the critical nature of having accessible and effective healthcare.

In this pivotal chapter, the exploration of why governments must prioritize the establishment of secure emergency health services becomes imperative. As individuals encounter moments of health crises where their bodies weaken, preventing them from pursuing self-healing practices, the reliance on professional medical assistance becomes indispensable. Highlighting the essence of timely and reliable emergency healthcare services can reinforce the notion that readiness and accessibility are fundamental pillars in safeguarding public health.

A thought-provoking introduction to this chapter could emphasize the intrinsic link between a well-functioning healthcare system and societal well-being. Governments hold the key to unlocking the potential for individuals to access emergency health services promptly and efficiently. Understanding that the ability to seek urgent medical help is a vital lifeline underscores the necessity for robust government initiatives aimed at bolstering emergency healthcare infrastructure.

Diving into the complexities of healthcare delivery, the chapter's introduction could shed light on the interconnected web of resources, personnel, and technology required to ensure the seamless provision of emergency health services. By unraveling the intricate tapestry that underpins emergency healthcare systems, the narrative can underscore the meticulous planning and continuous improvement efforts mandated for a resilient and secure healthcare framework.

As the canvas of healthcare landscapes evolves, the 9th chapter could set the stage for an insightful discussion on the evolving nature of emergency health services. Governments grapple with the dynamic challenges posed by emerging health threats, natural disasters, and pandemics, necessitating a constant reevaluation of strategies to fortify the resilience of emergency healthcare systems. By acknowledging the ever-changing healthcare landscape, the chapter can advocate for agile and adaptable government interventions to safeguard public health in times of crisis.

Within the narrative arc of this chapter, a poignant portrayal of the human impact of secure emergency health services can resonate deeply with readers. Highlighting real-life stories of individuals who have benefited from timely medical interventions can serve as a compelling testimony to the pivotal role emergency healthcare plays in saving lives and preserving well-being. By weaving these narratives into the fabric of the chapter's introduction, a profound emotional connection can be forged, reinforcing the urgency of securing robust emergency health services.

Expounding on the notion that everyone deserves equal access to emergency health services, the introduction could advocate for policies and initiatives that aim to bridge gaps in healthcare disparities. Governments bear the responsibility of ensuring that vulnerable populations, marginalized communities, and underserved regions have equitable access to emergency healthcare, thereby upholding the principles of social justice and healthcare equity. By championing inclusivity and accessibility in emergency healthcare, governments can pave the way towards a healthier and more equitable society.

Engaging in a discourse on the economic implications of secure emergency health services, the introduction could delve into the cost-effectiveness and long-term benefits of investing in robust healthcare infrastructures. By elucidating the economic rationale behind prioritizing emergency healthcare, the narrative can underscore that proactive investments in health systems yield dividends in terms of improved public health outcomes, enhanced workforce productivity, and reduced healthcare expenditures. Embracing a holistic perspective on the economic value of emergency health services, the chapter can advocate for prudent government expenditures that yield substantial returns in safeguarding public health.

Amidst the prevailing global challenges posed by health emergencies and pandemics, the chapter's introduction could emphasize the imperative of building resilient and adaptable emergency healthcare systems. Governments play a pivotal role in fostering collaboration, preparedness, and innovation in healthcare delivery, ensuring that emergency health services remain agile and responsive to emerging threats and crises. Harnessing the power of technology, data, and interdisciplinary partnerships, governments can lead the charge in fortifying emergency healthcare infrastructures to meet the evolving needs of society.

In conclusion, the introductory paragraph of the 9th chapter of my book holds the potential to ignite a dialogue on the intrinsic role governments play in securing emergency health services for all. By painting a vivid portrait of the critical importance of timely and reliable healthcare interventions in moments of crisis, the narrative can advocate for proactive government actions aimed at fortifying emergency healthcare systems. Through a multifaceted exploration of the social, economic, and human dimensions of emergency health services, the chapter can resonate with readers, compelling them to reflect on the indispensable nature of accessible and quality healthcare in safeguarding public well-being.

Chapter Ten: Empowering Health Autonomy: Navigating Wellness Through Online Resources

In the 10th chapter of my book, a profound exploration into the significance of leveraging internet resources for individuals aspiring to become self-sufficient in managing their health and well-being through self-education becomes the focal point. The narrative could delve into the transformative power of online platforms, particularly e-books and other digital resources, in equipping individuals with the knowledge and tools necessary to embark on a journey of self-healing and self-care. By illuminating the role of the internet as a gateway to becoming a 'Doctor to oneself,' the chapter sets the stage for an empowering discourse on the democratization of healthcare knowledge and the empowerment of individuals in taking charge of their own health destinies.

Delving deeper into the implications of individuals harnessing online resources to navigate the complexities of healthcare, the chapter's introduction could shed light on the paradigm shift underway in traditional notions of medical authority. By advocating for a model of empowerment and self-reliance in health management, the narrative challenges conventional hierarchies within the healthcare system and encourages individuals to embrace a proactive and informed approach to their well-being. In doing so, the chapter underscores the revolutionary potential of internet-based education in reshaping the dynamics of healthcare delivery and consumption.

Through a nuanced exploration of the intersection between online learning and healthcare autonomy, the introduction could illuminate the symbiotic relationship between individuals' self-education efforts and the broader imperative of enhancing healthcare security systems. By equipping individuals with the knowledge and skills to make informed health decisions through online resources, governments stand to benefit from a populace that is better equipped to navigate health challenges effectively and adopt preventive healthcare practices. This virtuous cycle of empowerment and wellness not only fosters individual resilience but also contributes to the collective health and security of society at large.

Emphasizing the far-reaching implications of individuals assuming agency over their health through online education, the chapter's introduction could underscore the potential for governments to streamline and simplify healthcare delivery systems. By promoting self-education initiatives that equip individuals with the know-how to proactively manage their health, governments can foster a culture of wellness that reduces the burden on traditional healthcare institutions and resources. This shift towards preventative and self-directed healthcare not only alleviates strain on the healthcare system but also engenders a sense of health freedom and self-empowerment among the populace.

In engendering a dialogue on the value proposition of online learning in healthcare literacy, the introduction could advocate for policies and initiatives that promote widespread access to digital health resources. By democratizing knowledge and information on health and wellness through e-books and online platforms, governments can bridge the gap in healthcare disparities and ensure that individuals from all walks of life have equal opportunities to become knowledgeable and conscientious 'Doctors to themselves.' This inclusivity and accessibility in health education lay the foundation for a society that is not only physically healthy but also empowered to make informed decisions about their well-being.

Within the narrative arc of this chapter, a poignant portrayal of the transformative potential of internet-based education in health management can resonate deeply with readers. By weaving together narratives of individuals who have successfully journeyed towards self-healing and self-care through online resources, the chapter can inspire and empower others to embark on a similar path of health autonomy. These stories of empowerment and resilience underscore the liberating impact of online learning in healthcare and reinforce the idea that becoming a genuine Doctor for oneself is both achievable and empowering.

Articulating the manifold benefits of individuals embracing online resources for health self-management, the introduction could advocate for a paradigm shift towards a more holistic and integrated approach to wellness. By encouraging individuals to supplement their healthcare journey with digital tools and educational resources, governments lay the groundwork for a society that is proactive, resilient, and empowered in matters of health. This holistic model of health empowerment not only fosters individual well-being but also contributes to the creation of a community that is attuned to the principles of self-care and health freedom.

Amidst the evolving landscape of digital health technologies and online platforms, the chapter's introduction could underscore the imperative of governments to adapt their security systems to safeguard individuals navigating online health resources. By prioritizing cybersecurity measures and regulatory frameworks that protect the integrity and privacy of health information shared online, governments can create a safe and secure environment for individuals to engage in self-education and self-care practices. This commitment to creating a trusted digital ecosystem for health empowerment underscores governments' role as enablers of health freedom and privacy in the digital age.

The introductory paragraphs of the 10th chapter of my book lay the groundwork for a compelling narrative on the transformative potential of online resources in empowering individuals to become self-sufficient 'Doctors to themselves.' By charting a course towards health autonomy and self-empowerment through digital education, the narrative advocates for a future where individuals are active participants in their health journeys and where governments play a vital role in fostering a culture of health freedom and resilience.

In the 10th chapter of my book, the focus shifts towards the transformative power of utilizing online resources, such as e-books and various online platforms, to empower individuals in the pursuit of self-education towards becoming their own health advocates and "Doctors to themselves". This chapter explores the significance of leveraging the vast information available on the internet to enhance one's knowledge and understanding of health-related topics, bridging the gap between traditional medical expertise and accessible self-care practices. By delving into the realm of digital learning and virtual resources, individuals are introduced to a wealth of knowledge that can shape their journey towards achieving a deeper sense of autonomy and self-sufficiency in matters of health and wellness.

As individuals navigate the boundless expanse of online repositories containing valuable health information, the 10th chapter delves into the advantages of harnessing these resources to cultivate a holistic approach to self-care and well-being. By tapping into digital platforms that offer insights on preventive measures, treatment options, and lifestyle modifications, individuals can equip themselves with the tools needed to take charge of their health destinies. Embracing the notion of self-education through online resources fosters a sense of agency and empowerment, enabling individuals to make informed decisions regarding their health and well-being.

Within the narrative of this chapter, an exploration of the role of governments in facilitating safe and user-friendly pathways for individuals to access online health resources unfolds. Governments can play a pivotal role in advocating for digital literacy, promoting ethical standards in online health content, and fostering secure platforms that uphold privacy and data protection. By creating an environment that supports individuals in navigating the vast digital landscape of health information, governments can contribute to the promotion of health freedom and empowerment, ensuring that individuals can make informed choices regarding their health without compromising on safety or authenticity.

Through an examination of the potential benefits of utilizing online resources for self-education in healthcare, the 10th chapter sheds light on how this approach can foster a sense of personal responsibility and accountability in health management. By encouraging individuals to engage with online materials that enhance their understanding of medical concepts, treatment modalities, and preventive strategies, the narrative underscores the pivotal role of self-education in promoting holistic well-being. Empowering individuals to proactively engage with their health through digital means not only cultivates a sense of ownership over one's well-being but also instills a proactive mindset towards health promotion and disease prevention.

Delving deeper into the transformative potential of online learning in healthcare, the chapter elucidates how individuals can leverage digital resources to complement traditional medical expertise and interventions. By assimilating knowledge from reputable e-books, online courses, and informational websites, individuals can broaden their understanding of complex health issues, explore alternative healing modalities, and gain insights into self-care practices that align with their unique needs and preferences. Integrating digital learning into the healthcare journey can serve as a catalyst for individuals to augment their health literacy, cultivate resilience in managing health challenges, and explore personalized approaches to well-being that resonate with their values and beliefs.

An examination of the symbiotic relationship between individual empowerment and governmental support in the realm of online health education takes center stage in the 10th chapter. Governments can champion initiatives that promote digital health literacy, encourage the dissemination of evidence-based health information, and enhance the accessibility of online resources for diverse populations. By fostering collaboration between healthcare professionals, technology experts, and policymakers, governments can pave the way for the development of user-friendly platforms that empower individuals to navigate the digital healthcare landscape with confidence and efficacy. Embracing a collaborative approach to advancing online health education can cultivate a culture of health independence and choice, enabling individuals to forge their unique paths towards optimal well-being.

Expounding on the notion that online self-education can serve as a gateway to personal transformation and empowerment, the 10th chapter advocates for a paradigm shift in how individuals perceive and engage with healthcare information. By embracing digital platforms as tools for self-discovery, learning, and growth, individuals can transcend traditional barriers to healthcare access, embark on a journey of self-empowerment, and cultivate a deeper connection to their health and vitality. Harnessing the power of online resources to become one's own health advocate not only enriches the individual's health journey but also contributes to the collective effort of building a society that values health freedom and self-determination.

Within the context of this chapter, the narrative explores the multifaceted benefits of integrating online learning into the fabric of healthcare delivery and wellness promotion. By leveraging e-books, informational websites, virtual seminars, and interactive platforms, individuals can explore diverse perspectives on health, wellness, and healing modalities, expanding their horizons and fostering a culture of continuous learning and self-improvement. Embracing the democratization of health information through online channels provides individuals with the opportunity to tailor their healthcare experiences, experiment with self-care practices, and embark on a transformative journey towards holistic well-being.

In the 10th chapter of my book, a compelling narrative unfolds, shedding light on the significance of leveraging online resources, particularly e-books, to empower individuals in becoming self-sufficient in managing their health. The chapter delves into the transformative potential of utilizing internet-based platforms and digital tools to equip individuals with the knowledge and skills needed to navigate their health journey independently. By advocating for the accessibility and democratization of healthcare information through online resources, the narrative underscores how individuals can effectively educate themselves to a level where they can essentially become their own doctors, albeit in a responsible and informed manner.

Central to the discourse is the notion that online platforms offer a plethora of e-books and resources that can serve as valuable educational tools for individuals aspiring to deepen their understanding of health and wellness. By emphasizing the role of self-directed learning and continuous education, the chapter highlights how digital resources can bridge the gap between traditional healthcare systems and the empowered individual seeking to take charge of their well-being. Through the democratization of knowledge and information, individuals can embark on a journey of self-empowerment, equipping themselves with the necessary tools to make informed decisions about their health.

The chapter explores how embracing digital resources and online platforms can enhance health literacy and promote a culture of preventive care. By encouraging individuals to engage with e-books and online materials that offer insights into key health concepts, disease prevention strategies, and lifestyle interventions, the narrative underscores how knowledge dissemination can empower individuals to proactively manage their health. This emphasis on preventive care not only fosters a sense of personal responsibility but also underscores the intrinsic link between knowledge and wellness.

Crucially, the chapter advocates for governments to recognize the pivotal role of digital health literacy in promoting public health outcomes and advancing societal well-being. By facilitating access to reputable online resources and educational platforms, governments can empower individuals to make informed decisions about their health, thereby reducing the reliance on traditional healthcare systems for basic healthcare needs. In doing so, governments can foster a culture of health independence, where individuals are equipped with the knowledge and tools needed to address their health concerns proactively.

The narrative underscores how the utilization of online resources can help mitigate the financial barriers that often hinder individuals from accessing quality healthcare services. By providing individuals with access to free or low-cost e-books and digital resources on healthcare, governments can democratize health information and promote health equity. No individual should face the dire consequence of being unable to afford essential healthcare services simply because of financial constraints. Empowering individuals with the knowledge and skills to care for themselves through online resources represents a significant step towards creating a more equitable and inclusive healthcare landscape.

Drawing a poignant parallel between access to online health resources and the fundamental right to health, the chapter advocates for a paradigm shift in how healthcare is perceived and accessed. The narrative challenges the traditional notion that becoming a genuine doctor for oneself requires formal education or financial means. Through the democratization of health information via online platforms, individuals can transcend barriers to traditional healthcare and embrace a model of self-care and empowerment. This shift towards health autonomy not only empowers individuals but also fosters a sense of agency and control over one's well-being.

Additionally, the chapter delves into the concept of health freedom and the profound impact that digital health resources can have on enhancing individual autonomy and decision-making. By equipping individuals with the knowledge and tools to navigate their health journey independently, online resources can catalyze a paradigm shift towards a healthcare model that prioritizes personal agency and informed choice. In essence, the chapter underscores how embracing digital platforms for health education allows individuals to chart their own path towards wellness, free from external constraints or dependencies on traditional healthcare systems.

The chapter advocates for a symbiotic relationship between individuals leveraging online resources for self-care and governments creating simple and safe avenues for health promotion. By promoting the use of digital health resources as a means to enhance personal health literacy, governments can lay the groundwork for a society where individuals are empowered to take charge of their well-being. This collaborative approach between individuals and governments not only fosters a culture of health independence but also positions digital platforms as invaluable tools for advancing public health agendas and promoting population well-being.

The narrative underscores how the convergence of technology and healthcare can revolutionize the way individuals approach their health and well-being. By embracing online resources and digital tools for self-education, individuals can transcend geographical barriers, time constraints, and financial limitations that may impede access to traditional healthcare services. This shift towards a digitally empowered healthcare paradigm holds the promise of democratizing health information, promoting health equity, and fostering a society where individuals have the autonomy and knowledge to lead healthier lives.

In the 10th chapter of my book, the focus on the intersection of internet usage, personal healthcare empowerment, and government security measures propels the narrative into a realm where the democratization of medical knowledge through e-books and online resources becomes a pivotal catalyst for individual agency in assuming the role of self-doctoring. By illuminating the significance of accessing reliable healthcare information online, the chapter elevates the discourse on how governments can harness technology to foster a populace adept at safeguarding their well-being.

The chapter delves into the transformative potential of leveraging internet-based resources to equip individuals with the necessary insights and tools to embark on a journey of self-education in healthcare matters. The accessibility of e-books and online healthcare resources presents an unparalleled opportunity for people to expand their knowledge base, thereby creating a path towards becoming informed and discerning guardians of their own health. This paradigm shift not only empowers individuals but also prompts governments to consider the implications of a populace with the capability to navigate their health journey with newfound autonomy.

Central to the narrative of this chapter is the notion of enhancing public health resilience through widespread access to credible health information available online. By emphasizing the invaluable role of digital resources in fostering a culture of health literacy and proactive self-care, the narrative underscores the inherent benefits of individuals embracing their roles as proactive stewards of their well-being. Coupled with the government's commitment to cultivating simplified and secure pathways for individuals to access online healthcare information, this symbiotic relationship epitomizes a proactive stance towards fortifying the foundations of health freedom.

Within the chapter's discourse, an impassioned plea emerges for the assurance that no individual should face dire health consequences due to a lack of financial resources to access essential care. By equipping individuals with the knowledge and tools to engage in self-doctoring practices through online resources, the narrative asserts an inherent commitment to mitigating circumstances where individuals are left vulnerable to health crises due to financial constraints. In doing so, the chapter exhorts governments to consider the imperative of embracing digital health empowerment as a means to realize the fundamental right to health and well-being for all.

The interconnectivity of internet-enabled health literacy, government security protocols, and personal health freedom forms the cornerstone of the chapter's thematic narrative. Advocating for the symbiotic relationship between individuals utilizing digital resources for self-doctoring and governments fostering secure online avenues for health information, the chapter underscore the reciprocal advantages inherent in embracing this synergy. In the quest for enriching health freedom, the narrative articulates the pivotal role of governments in aligning security systems to facilitate a seamless and protected online healthcare landscape, thereby empowering individuals to navigate their health journey with confidence and assurance.

The chapter's exploration extends beyond the individual sphere, delving into how the proliferation of e-books and online healthcare resources can be harnessed to bolster population health resilience on a broader scale. By embracing the potential of internet-enabled health education, governments can catalyze a paradigm shift towards a more empowered and knowledgeable citizenry capable of proactive health management. This not only cultivates a populace well-versed in pre-emptive health measures but also serves as a cornerstone for governments to orchestrate comprehensive health policies aligned with the needs of an increasingly health-conscious populace.

Amid the tides of change reshaping healthcare landscapes, the chapter emphasizes the profound impact of embracing digital health literacy as a catalyst for individual and collective health emancipation. Through an enriching mosaic of narratives and insights, the chapter highlights how the seamless deployment of secure online healthcare resources can bridge the divide between conventional healthcare delivery and the burgeoning realm of digital self-doctoring. This convergence not only empowers individuals to access a wealth of healthcare knowledge but also presents governments with a unique opportunity to curate and optimize secure digital conduits for the dissemination of reliable health information.

The underlying thrust of the chapter pivots around the fundamental belief that no individual should be condemned to suffering or peril due to an inability to access essential healthcare. By championing the ethos of personal health empowerment through digital resources, the narrative champions a vision where individuals become architects of their health destiny, unperturbed by financial barriers that often impede access to healthcare. Governments, attuned to this pervasive shift, are implored to pivot their security measures to not only safeguard online health data but also foster an environment where individuals can avidly pursue their health aspirations with comprehensive support and protection.

The 10th chapter of my book resonates with an impassioned plea for the integration of internet-enabled health education, government security protocols, and individual health freedom in a symphony aimed at transfiguring the healthcare landscape. By unraveling the transformative potential of digital health literacy, the narrative envisions a future where individuals are emboldened to embrace their roles as guardians of their well-being, thus endeavoring to manifest a society where no one's health is compromised due to financial limitations. The chapter serves as a clarion call to governments to navigate the evolving contours of healthcare empowerment and security, thereby fostering a terrain where individuals can traverse their health journey with a sense of liberty, assurance, and resilience.

In the 10th chapter of my book, the focus on the crucial role of security systems in the context of individuals using the internet to educate themselves and access resources to become self-empowered in healthcare is paramount. Within this chapter, the exploration of how the government's security efforts intersect with the democratization of healthcare knowledge and access to online resources can shed light on the transformative potential of digital platforms in fostering health freedom and autonomy.

As the digital landscape increasingly shapes the dissemination of medical knowledge and resources, the chapter's conclusion has the opportunity to underscore the pivotal responsibility of governments in ensuring the security and reliability of online healthcare information. By emphasizing the importance of robust security systems, the narrative can advocate for a safe and trustworthy online environment, enabling individuals to access accurate and comprehensive healthcare knowledge without compromising the integrity of the information.

The culmination of the 10th chapter presents an apt occasion to emphasize the profound societal impact of individuals harnessing digital resources to become knowledgeable about self-care and preventive healthcare measures. Governments play a critical role in bolstering the security infrastructure of online platforms, thereby facilitating safe and uninhibited access to healthcare resources. Emphasizing the notion that no individual should face the risk of poor health outcomes due to a lack of access to reliable healthcare information reinforces the urgent need for secure digital avenues for self-education in healthcare.

The conclusion paragraph of the 10th chapter can articulate how the proliferation of online healthcare resources, coupled with stringent security measures, aligns with the broader goal of enhancing public health freedoms. By empowering individuals to become "doctors to themselves" through reputable online resources, governments can catalyze a paradigm shift towards proactive and preventive healthcare practices. This, in turn, can lead to a society where individuals are equipped with the knowledge and tools to actively participate in their own well-being, ensuring that preventable illnesses and health concerns do not burgeon into unmanageable crises.

Importantly, the narrative within the chapter's conclusion could stress the ethical imperative for governments to facilitate secure and accessible avenues for individuals to attain healthcare knowledge online. In a global landscape where financial barriers can impede access to traditional healthcare services, advocating for secure online resources as a means of self-education in healthcare aligns with the fundamental principle that no individual should face dire health consequences due to financial constraints. Emphasizing the linkage between secure online healthcare resources, health equity, and the universal right to wellness can inspire collective action towards creating a future where individuals are not bound by financial limitations in pursuit of good health.

Moreover, the chapter's conclusion serves as a platform to expound on the transformative potential of secure online healthcare education in fostering a culture of informed decision-making and proactive health management. Governments stand to benefit from the emergence of a digitally savvy, health-conscious populace, as individuals empowered with accurate medical knowledge can contribute to alleviating the burden on traditional healthcare systems. By advocating for secure digital platforms as enablers of self-empowerment in healthcare, the chapter's conclusion can underscore the symbiotic relationship between government security measures and the cultivation of a proactive, health-empowered society.

In closing, the 10th chapter's conclusion can encapsulate the narrative's advocacy for secure online healthcare resources as a conduit for democratizing health knowledge and fostering health freedom. By amplifying the imperative of robust security systems, the narrative underscores the pivotal role of governments in safeguarding access to reliable and accurate healthcare information online. Embracing a vision where no individual confronts dire health circumstances due to a lack of opportunities for self-education in healthcare, the chapter's conclusion champions a future where online healthcare resources serve as pathways to wellness and longevity, irrespective of financial constraints.

Chapter Eleven: Guiding Light: Navigating Healthcare Insecurities and Embracing Health Freedom

In crafting the introductory paragraphs for the 11th chapter of my book, the focus shifts towards the critical significance of the book's content in providing a guiding light for individuals navigating healthcare insecurities in various contexts. The chapter sets the stage for elucidating how the comprehensive insights shared throughout the book can serve as a supportive resource for readers seeking discipline-specific healthcare services, irrespective of their social or economic status.

The 11th chapter delves into the essential role of this book as a beacon of knowledge and empowerment for individuals confronting health care uncertainties across diverse terrains. By underscoring how the book's guidance can offer solace and direction in times of need, the narrative underscores the far-reaching impact of equipping readers with the tools and information needed to navigate complex health challenges effectively.

At its core, the introductory paragraphs of this chapter can underline the inclusive nature of the book's content, transcending socio-economic boundaries to cater to individuals from all walks of life. The narrative emphasizes how the book's guidance can provide invaluable support to people from varied backgrounds, underscoring the universal need for discipline-specific healthcare services and the transformative power of accessible knowledge in fostering well-being.

Moreover, the chapter's introduction can illuminate how the insights and wisdom curated within the book can catalyze positive change not only at the individual level but also on a broader societal scale. By highlighting how the book's guidance aligns with the vision of creating simple and secure avenues for individuals to attain health freedom, the narrative underscores the ripple effect this knowledge can have in shaping public health policies and initiatives led by governments.

In a world where health disparities persist and access to quality healthcare remains a challenge for many, the introductory paragraphs of the 11th chapter underscore the pivotal role of the book in bridging these gaps and championing health equity. By advocating for the book as a tool that empowers individuals to take charge of their health needs in a disciplined and informed manner, the narrative positions itself as a catalyst for change, urging for a more inclusive and accessible healthcare landscape that transcends societal barriers.

The introduction to this chapter lays the groundwork for exploring how the book's insights can foster a culture of self-reliance and proactive health management among readers. By emphasizing the book's potential to guide individuals in making informed decisions about their health regardless of their social standing, the narrative underscores the transformative impact of equipping people with the knowledge and resources needed to navigate the complexities of healthcare with confidence and agency.

Within the fabric of the introductory paragraphs, there lies a narrative thread that weaves together the themes of empowerment, inclusivity, and governmental responsibility in shaping a healthcare ecosystem that prioritizes individual needs and health freedom. By positioning the book as a catalyst for both personal and societal transformation, the narrative underscores the

interconnected nature of individual well-being and the broader health landscape, advocating for collaborative efforts between individuals and governments to create a healthier and more equitable society.

Embracing the ethos of knowledge dissemination and empowerment, the introduction to the 11th chapter advocates for the book's instrumental role in sparking conversations, driving forward policy changes, and inspiring collective action towards a future where healthcare is a universal right accessible to all. By shining a spotlight on the book's potential to inspire positive change and catalyze grassroots movements for health justice, the narrative frames the dissemination of healthcare knowledge as a means to foster empathy, understanding, and solidarity among diverse communities.

The introductory paragraphs of the 11th chapter herald the transformative potential of the book as a guidepost for individuals navigating health care insecurities and seeking discipline-specific healthcare services. By emphasizing the book's accessibility and universal relevance, the narrative positions itself as a tool for empowerment and enlightenment, transcending societal barriers to champion health freedom for all. By advocating for the book's role in sparking positive change at personal, communal, and governmental levels, the narrative lays the foundation for a discourse on the symbiotic relationship between knowledge, empowerment, and societal well-being in the realm of healthcare.

In the 11th chapter of my book, the focus on the importance of creating such a comprehensive guide for healthcare self-empowerment resonates deeply with the fundamental need for inclusive and accessible healthcare knowledge. This book serves as a supportive and instructive tool, one that has the potential to alleviate health care insecurities for individuals, irrespective of their socio-economic background. By highlighting the wide-reaching impact of this guide in equipping individuals with discipline-wise healthcare guidance, the narrative underscores its potential to transcend barriers and empower individuals to take charge of their well-being.

The 11th chapter's significance lies in its articulation of how this book can provide invaluable support to individuals navigating through health care insecurities, whether they arise from financial limitations, geographical constraints, or systemic disparities. By envisaging the far-reaching impact of this guide in bridging gaps in accessible healthcare education and resources, the narrative underscores its potential to be a lifeline for those in need. It is through the comprehensive and discipline-wise healthcare guidance encapsulated within this book that individuals from all walks of life can find solace and empowerment, transcending limitations and fostering a culture of health freedom.

The fundamental premise of this book's significance lies in its potential to empower governments and policymakers to architect simple, secure, and equitable avenues for individuals to access healthcare knowledge and resources. The comprehensive nature of this guide underscores its ability to serve as a blueprint for innovative governmental initiatives aimed at democratizing health education and ensuring that all individuals, regardless of their social or economic standing, can access discipline-wise healthcare guidance. By embracing this guide as a catalyst for reform, governments can steer towards a future where health freedom is not a privilege but an inherent right for every individual.

At the heart of the 11th chapter lies the vision of a society where individuals, irrespective of their class or background, are equipped with the knowledge and discipline-wise guidance necessary to make informed healthcare decisions. This book stands as a testament to the ethos of inclusivity and accessibility, fostering a reality where healthcare education transcends socio-economic barriers and empowers every individual to attain the highest standard of well-being. Recognizing the transformative potential of this guide, the narrative underscores its pivotal role in cultivating a society where access to high-quality healthcare knowledge becomes an unalienable right, not contingent upon one's economic or social status.

Furthermore, the 11th chapter underscores the book's role in underscoring the urgent need for sustainable and equitable healthcare solutions. By incorporating discipline-wise healthcare guidance that is tailored to meet the diverse needs of individuals from varying backgrounds, the narrative advocates for a future where healthcare services are not only accessible but also sustainable and adaptive. Through the dissemination of this thoughtful and comprehensive guide, the potential to shape a future where healthcare delivery is both simple and secure becomes within reach, igniting a transformative shift towards a society where health freedom is an inalienable aspect of daily life.

Embracing the far-reaching scope of this book's influence, the 11th chapter underscores the pivotal role it can play in inspiring collective action towards redefining the paradigm of health freedom. By envisioning a future where individuals are equipped with the discipline-wise healthcare guidance encapsulated within this guide, the narrative emphasizes the transformative potential to foster a culture of proactive health management and informed decision-making. Through the lens of this comprehensive guide, the narrative paints a compelling vision of a society where individuals are not merely passive recipients of healthcare but active participants in their well-being, thereby transcending class-based disparities and fostering a culture of universal health freedom.

The 11th chapter serves as a poignant testimony to the transformative potential of this comprehensive guide for healthcare empowerment. By emphasizing its ability to alleviate health care insecurities, embrace individuals from all social strata, and inspire governmental innovation towards health equity, the narrative underscores the profound significance of this book. Through the comprehensive discipline-wise healthcare guidance it encapsulates, the guide heralds a future where health freedom is not a privilege but a fundamental right, fostering a society where every individual can live a life full of health freedom, unbounded by class or circumstance.

In the 11th chapter, it is essential to articulate the significance of creating such a book that offers comprehensive guidance in navigating health care insecurities. This book stands to serve as a beacon of support for individuals encountering health care uncertainties across various contexts, offering insights and strategies to foster resilience and informed decision-making. By illuminating the importance of this resource, the narrative can underscore its potential as a supportive tool for individuals seeking structured and disciplined health care services, irrespective of their social or economic standing.

Through a nuanced exploration of the value of this book, the 11th chapter can emphasize how it serves as a foundational resource for individuals who may encounter challenges in accessing quality health care. Whether facing financial constraints, geographical barriers, or systemic disparities, the book's guidance can serve as a roadmap for individuals navigating the labyrinth of health care insecurities, empowering them to make informed choices and advocate for their well-being. Positioning the book as a leveller that transcends social classes, the chapter can convey its potential as a unifying force in fostering comprehensive and discipline-wise health care practices.

The chapter can underscore the book's capacity to catalyze the creation of simple and secure health care pathways, harmonizing with the broader vision of fostering health freedom for all. By delineating the ways in which the book equips individuals with the knowledge and agency to navigate health care systems, the narrative can advocate for the transformative potential of this resource in enabling individuals to lead lives imbued with health autonomy and well-being. Embracing a vision where individuals are empowered to proactively engage with their health care needs, the chapter can underscore the symbiotic relationship between the book's guidance and the realization of health freedom for people across diverse walks of life.

The elucidation of the book's pivotal role in fostering discipline-wise health care practices can resonate deeply with readers, underscoring the intrinsic value of informed decision-making and proactive health management. By imbuing individuals with a comprehensive understanding of health care disciplines and strategies, the book transcends borders and barriers, serving as a compass for individuals navigating the vast and often complex terrain of health care. This depiction underscores the universal relevance of the book's guidance, emphasizing its capacity to guide people from various backgrounds towards cultivating health-conscious disciplines and practices.

In emphasizing the significance of this book, the chapter can also spotlight the potential for governments to leverage its insights in creating streamlined and inclusive health care pathways. By positioning the book as a valuable resource capable of informing governmental policies and initiatives, the narrative can advocate for the collaborative role of governments in fostering secure and accessible health care systems. Illustrating how the book's guidance aligns with the broader imperative of advancing health freedom, the chapter can underscore its capacity to inform and inspire government efforts in creating simple, effective, and safe health care platforms for all.

The chapter's exploration of the book's significance can extend to articulating its ability to serve as a cornerstone in the cultivation of a culture of disciplined and informed health care practices. By underscoring how the book's guidance can permeate diverse strata of society, nurturing a collective ethos of health consciousness, the narrative underscores its potential to drive a societal shift towards disciplined and proactive health care management. Embracing a vision where individuals across various classes and communities are equipped with the tools and knowledge to engage with their health care needs, the chapter can advocate for the book's role as a catalyst in fostering a culture of health empowerment and collective well-being.

The 11th chapter's poignant exploration of the significance of this book can resonate as a testament to its transformative potential in addressing health care insecurities and fostering health freedom. By amplifying its role as a supportive guide for individuals navigating health care challenges, irrespective of their backgrounds, the narrative underscores its capacity to transcend social classes and empower individuals with discipline-wise health care strategies. Embracing a vision where the book sparks a societal shift towards proactive health management and informed decision-making, the chapter champions its intrinsic value as a pathway towards a future where health autonomy and well-being are accessible to all.

Chapter Twelve: Futuristic Healthcare Horizons: Governments Leading the Way with Advanced Laboratory Services and High-Tech Tools

In the 12th chapter of my book, the spotlight shines brightly on the pivotal role of governments in advancing state-of-the-art laboratory services and high-tech healthcare tools. This thoughtful exploration propels the narrative into the realm of futuristic healthcare innovation, emphasizing the profound impact of cutting-edge laboratory technology and healthcare tools on individuals' ability to proactively engage in self-care and education. The chapter positions the convergence of advanced health tech and accessible online resources as a gateway to empowering individuals to assume greater agency in managing their well-being.

As the chapter unfolds, the compelling narrative underscores the intrinsic link between the accessibility of advanced laboratory services and high-tech healthcare tools and the democratization of medical knowledge. By acknowledging the transformative power of digital platforms and e-books in disseminating healthcare information, the narrative advocates for the synergy between technological advancements and individual empowerment. This fusion empowers individuals to harness the vast wealth of online resources to cultivate a deeper understanding of their health, effectively assuming the role of self-guided "Doctors" in their healthcare journey.

Delving deeper into the profound influence of cutting-edge laboratory services and high-tech healthcare tools, the chapter elucidates how the convergence of technology and healthcare not only augments individuals' ability to access critical health information but also lays the groundwork for proactive health management. The narrative advocates for governments to spearhead initiatives aimed at democratizing access to advanced laboratory services and healthcare tools, envisioning a future where individuals can leverage innovative diagnostics and digital health solutions to make informed decisions about their well-being.

A poignant exploration of the societal ramifications underpins this chapter's narrative, painting a vivid picture of the far-reaching implications of individuals being denied access to essential healthcare due to financial constraints. The harrowing reality of individuals facing life-threatening health conditions without the means to afford medical care serves as a stark reminder of the urgent need for governments to proactively embrace initiatives that advance accessible and cost-effective healthcare technologies. The chapter champions the fundamental principle that no individual should face the prospect of mortality simply due to financial barriers to healthcare access, articulating a poignant call to action for governments to prioritize the development of inclusive health tech solutions.

The narrative arc unfolds to underscore the symbiotic relationship between advanced laboratory services, high-tech healthcare tools, and the pursuit of health freedom. By illuminating the potential of cutting-edge diagnostics and technology-driven healthcare interventions in enabling individuals to take ownership of their health, the narrative envisions a world where individuals are empowered to proactively engage in wellness-seeking behaviors and make informed healthcare decisions. Governments are positioned as pivotal agents in shaping a future where health freedom is not an elusive privilege but an attainable right for all individuals, grounded in the seamless access to transformative healthcare technologies.

Extending beyond individual empowerment, the chapter transcends to underscore the profound societal benefits that stem from governments prioritizing advancements in laboratory services and healthcare technologies. The narrative articulates how the pursuit of cutting-edge innovations lays the foundation for a healthcare landscape characterized by preventive interventions, early disease detection, and personalized health management. By championing this paradigm shift towards proactive and personalized healthcare, the chapter advocates for governments to embrace visionary policies and investments that foster a culture of health empowerment and resilience.

The chapter weaves a compelling narrative that speaks to the imperative of advancing healthcare technologies to bridge the gap between diagnosis and action, underscoring the transformative potential of leveraging advanced laboratory services and high-tech healthcare tools. By facilitating the convergence of data-driven insights and actionable healthcare interventions, governments can not only equip individuals with the tools to make informed health decisions but also catalyze a paradigm shift towards preventive and proactive healthcare. The narrative underscores the profound societal value in cultivating a healthcare ecosystem where timely and accurate diagnostics seamlessly translate into tangible outcomes, thereby mitigating the burden of preventable illnesses and fostering a culture of health empowerment.

At its core, the chapter presents a resounding case for governments to harness the transformative potential of advanced laboratory services and high-tech healthcare tools as catalysts for shaping a healthcare landscape characterized by accessibility, efficacy, and health equity. The narrative emanates a clarion call for governments to spearhead initiatives that democratize access to cutting-edge diagnostics, therapeutic innovations, and digital health solutions, thereby transforming the paradigm of healthcare delivery from reactive to proactive. By embracing this visionary trajectory, governments can position themselves as champions of health freedom, engendering a society where individuals are empowered to navigate their health journeys with resilience, resourcefulness, and agency.

In the 12th chapter of my book, a profound exploration into the significance of governments focusing on developing state-of-the-art laboratory services and cutting-edge healthcare technologies emerges as a pivotal subject. By elucidating the critical role of advanced laboratory tools in tandem with high-tech healthcare devices, the narrative can illuminate how these innovations profoundly impact individuals' ability to access healthcare information and resources. Particularly in an era where individuals increasingly turn to the internet as a source of medical knowledge, the synergy between advanced technologies and accessible health information becomes paramount in empowering individuals to take charge of their health and well-being.

Delving into the realm of self-empowerment through digital resources, the chapter could underscore how the integration of best laboratory services and high-tech healthcare tools enhances individuals' capacity to educate themselves on healthcare practices. By leveraging e-books, online resources, and digital platforms, individuals can embark on a journey towards becoming well-informed and proactive in managing their health. Through fostering a culture of self-education and empowerment, governments can play a vital role in equipping individuals with the tools and knowledge needed to make informed healthcare decisions, irrespective of their financial resources.

Articulating the interconnectedness between technological advancements in healthcare and the democratization of medical knowledge, the chapter can shed light on how enhancing laboratory services and healthcare technologies facilitates individuals' pursuit of self-sufficiency in healthcare. By harnessing the potential of digital platforms and cutting-edge tools, individuals can access a wealth of medical information, diagnostic capabilities, and treatment options that were once exclusive to traditional healthcare settings. Enabling individuals to become their own 'doctors' through digital literacy and technological tools not only empowers them to take charge of their health but also mitigates barriers to healthcare access, including financial constraints.

In the context of healthcare equity and social justice, the discussion within the chapter could advocate for the imperative of ensuring that individuals do not face dire health consequences due to lack of financial resources. Governments, by investing in advanced laboratory services and high-tech healthcare tools, can pave the way for innovative solutions that bridge the gap between healthcare affordability and quality. No individual should be compelled to forgo necessary medical care or succumb to illness due to financial constraints. By bolstering technological advancements in healthcare, governments can create opportunities for individuals to seek cost-effective healthcare solutions and access vital health information in an inclusive and equitable manner.

Emphasizing the transformative potential of advanced healthcare technologies in facilitating comprehensive health management, the chapter could elucidate how individuals can benefit from a spectrum of health-enhancing tools, from diagnostic equipment to monitoring devices, in their pursuit of well-being. The integration of high-tech laboratory services and healthcare tools not only enhances preventive healthcare measures but also enables individuals to address health concerns proactively. By leveraging technological innovations, individuals can engage in early detection of health issues, real-time monitoring of vital signs, and personalized health interventions, thereby promoting a proactive approach to maintaining health and preventing diseases.

Unveiling the intrinsic link between advanced laboratory services, healthcare technologies, and people's quest for reliable health information, the chapter can highlight how individuals increasingly rely on digital resources and online platforms to access credible healthcare guidance. With the proliferation of online health resources, individuals have the opportunity to educate themselves on diverse health topics, explore treatment options, and learn about preventive measures. By aligning government efforts with the evolving landscape of digital healthcare resources, individuals can leverage technology to empower themselves with essential health knowledge, thereby fostering a culture of self-care and health literacy.

Envisioning a future where individuals can navigate healthcare complexities with confidence and autonomy, the chapter could underscore how advancing health tech tools and laboratory services can redefine the paradigm of healthcare accessibility and empowerment. By enabling individuals to harness digital resources and cutting-edge technologies, governments can facilitate a healthcare landscape where individuals are equipped to make informed decisions about their health with ease and precision. Empowering individuals to leverage high-tech solutions for health management not only enhances their quality of life but also cultivates a society where health freedom and self-determination are foundational principles.

In light of the transformative impact that advanced healthcare technologies can have on public health outcomes, the chapter could advocate for progressive government policies that prioritize innovation in healthcare delivery. Governments, through strategic investments in research, development, and implementation of state-of-the-art laboratory services and healthcare technologies, can steer society towards a future where healthcare is personalized, accessible, and efficient. By championing a culture of innovation and progress in healthcare, governments can harness the full potential of technology to revolutionize healthcare delivery, prevent unnecessary health disparities, and ensure that individuals have the tools they need to lead healthy and fulfilling lives.

Propelling the discourse towards a vision of healthcare inclusivity and empowerment, the chapter could illuminate how advancements in laboratory services and healthcare technologies pave the way for creating simple, safe, and accessible pathways for individuals to achieve health freedom. By amplifying the availability of digital health resources, promoting health literacy, and enhancing healthcare infrastructure, governments can empower individuals to make informed choices about their health without being hindered by financial constraints.

In the 12th chapter of my book, the pivotal discussion focuses on the significant importance for governments to allocate resources and efforts towards enhancing laboratory services and implementing state-of-the-art healthcare technologies. This emphasis on technological advancements in laboratory tools, as well as other healthcare technology, holds the potential to revolutionize the way individuals access and utilize medical information. The synergy between advanced laboratory services and cutting-edge healthcare tools facilitates the burgeoning trend of individuals leveraging the internet to empower themselves with knowledge, akin to becoming self-sufficient doctors through the vast array of online resources, including e-books and other educational materials. By accentuating the indispensable role of these technological advancements, the narrative underscores their pivotal contribution in allowing individuals to make informed health decisions, thereby promoting self-advocacy and autonomy in managing their well-being.

The development and integration of advanced laboratory and healthcare technologies epitomize a paradigm shift in the realm of self-directed healthcare. By elevating the accessibility and reliability of health information, individuals are empowered to seek out comprehensive understanding and make informed choices regarding their health and well-being. The intersection of modern laboratory services and cutting-edge healthcare tools not only facilitates self-education but also fosters a sense of health literacy, equipping individuals with the essential knowledge to navigate the complex healthcare landscape. Governments' prioritization of these technological advancements serves as a catalyst for democratizing healthcare, ensuring that individuals are not deprived of critical medical insights due to financial constraints.

The advancement of high-tech laboratory and healthcare tools emerges as a linchpin in addressing the pervasive issue of healthcare accessibility and affordability. With individuals increasingly relying on internet-based resources to self-educate and make informed healthcare decisions, the value of robust laboratory services and advanced healthcare technologies becomes even more pronounced. These advancements not only enable individuals to discern vital health insights but also facilitate the pursuit of streamlined, cost-effective medical solutions. The convergence of accessible medical information and technologically-advanced healthcare tools lays the groundwork for governments to create pathways for individuals to access quality, affordable healthcare, thus averting scenarios where financial constraints culminate in dire health outcomes.

Crucially, the advancement of laboratory and healthcare technologies serves as a cornerstone in forging health freedom for individuals. By enabling comprehensive access to critical health information and diagnostics, individuals are empowered to proactively engage in their well-being, thereby mitigating the dire consequences of lack of access to healthcare due to financial limitations. The intersection of progressive healthcare technologies and the burgeoning virtual repository of healthcare-related knowledge positions governments to cultivate an environment where individuals are equipped with the means to lead healthy, informed lives, irrespective of economic disparities. The deployment of sophisticated health technologies also aligns with the broader imperative of instilling a sense of personal agency and self-determination in individuals' healthcare journeys, effectively fostering a society where the specter of compromised health due to financial constraints is significantly mitigated.

The advancement of laboratory services and healthcare technologies aligns with the overarching endeavor to eradicate preventable health crises attributed to lack of access to medical resources. As individuals increasingly rely on the internet and digital platforms to access healthcare-related information, the need for reliable, cutting-edge laboratory services and healthcare technologies becomes paramount. This convergence not only catalyzes individuals' ability to access vital health insights but also lays the groundwork for the expeditious interpretation of health-related data and the formulation of informed medical decisions. Governments spearheading the integration of advanced healthcare technologies and laboratory services lay the robust groundwork for a healthcare landscape where individuals are empowered to avert preventable health crises and proactively manage their well-being through informed, data-driven healthcare decisions.

The alignment of forward-looking laboratory services and high-tech healthcare tools serves as a testament to the pivotal role of technology in augmenting healthcare self-advocacy and autonomy. The strategic investments in advancing laboratory and healthcare technologies bolster the arsenal of resources available to individuals as they embark on autonomous healthcare journeys. This amalgamation of technological advancements not only augments individuals' ability to self-educate and make informed health decisions but also demystifies the complexities of medical information, establishing a foundation for proactive health management. The synergistic integration of advanced healthcare technologies and laboratory services thus serves as a clarion call for governments to pioneer a healthcare landscape where individuals are fortified with the requisite tools and insights to unshackle themselves from the shackles of healthcare limitations driven by financial inadequacies.

The prudent pursuit of technological advancements in laboratory services and healthcare tools aligns with the paramount imperative of ensuring that no individual succumbs to adverse health outcomes directly linked to financial constraints. By fostering a healthcare environment where individuals harness the power of advanced technologies to assimilate crucial health information and make informed medical choices, the trajectory toward equitable healthcare access is decisively charted. The amalgamation of progressive laboratory services and high-tech healthcare tools serves as an exemplar of governments' unwavering commitment to engendering a healthcare landscape where individuals are equipped with the resources and autonomy to pursue proactive, well-informed healthcare decisions, thus obviating dire health outcomes precipitated by financial hurdles.

In the concluding chapter of my book, the emphasis on the critical importance of governments investing in cutting-edge laboratory services and high-tech healthcare tools resonates profoundly. By recognizing the transformative potential of advanced technologies in enhancing healthcare delivery and empowering individuals to take charge of their health, the narrative delves into the profound impact that innovative healthcare solutions can have on society as a whole. Governments stand at the nexus of driving forward progress in healthcare technology, paving the way for a future where individuals can leverage digital resources to become their own advocates for health and well-being.

As the narrative unfolds, one of the key takeaways lies in the pivotal role of technology in democratizing access to healthcare knowledge and resources. In an era where the internet serves as a vast repository of information and wisdom, individuals have the unprecedented opportunity to educate themselves on healthcare practices, conditions, and treatment options. By harnessing the power of e-books, online resources, and interactive platforms, people can embark on a journey of self-discovery and self-care, transforming themselves into informed participants in their own healthcare journeys. This paradigm shift underscores the profound significance of governments investing in state-of-the-art laboratory services and high-tech healthcare tools to catalyze this digital health revolution.

The narrative underscores the stark reality that financial constraints should not be a barrier preventing individuals from accessing life-saving healthcare. The vision of a world where no one succumbs to illness due to lack of financial resources to afford medical care underscores the urgency for governments to innovate and implement cost-effective solutions that ensure healthcare is a fundamental human right, not a privilege reserved for the wealthy. By advancing technology-driven healthcare tools, governments can bridge the gap between healthcare affordability and quality, guaranteeing that every individual has the opportunity to lead a healthy and fulfilling life, devoid of financial hardships impeding their access to essential medical services.

The symbiotic relationship between cutting-edge laboratory services, high-tech healthcare tools, and the empowerment of individuals to take charge of their health underpins the overarching theme of the chapter. By enabling people to harness the power of technology to make informed healthcare decisions and leverage the insights generated by modern laboratory services, governments set the stage for a paradigm shift in how healthcare is accessed, delivered, and personalized to individual needs. This confluence of advanced health technologies and digital literacy opens pathways for individuals to proactively manage their health, seek timely interventions, and engage in preventive practices that promote long-term well-being.

Furthermore, the chapter underscores the transformative potential of advancing healthcare technology beyond the confines of traditional healthcare settings. By integrating sophisticated laboratory services and high-tech healthcare tools into everyday life, governments can empower individuals to track their health metrics, monitor chronic conditions, and receive personalized insights that guide them towards healthier lifestyles. Harnessing the synergy between technology, data analytics, and healthcare expertise, governments can cultivate a culture of proactive health management, preventive care, and early intervention strategies that mitigate the burden of disease and promote longevity.

The narrative culminates in envisioning a future where governments lay the foundation for a healthcare ecosystem where individuals are not passive recipients of medical care but active participants in their health journeys. By fostering a culture of health literacy, digital empowerment, and accessibility to cutting-edge healthcare technologies, governments pave the way for a society where individuals are equipped with the knowledge, tools, and resources to navigate the complexities of health with confidence and autonomy. This transformative shift towards a proactive, preventive, and patient-centric healthcare model underscores the transformative power of governments investing in innovative laboratory services and high-tech healthcare tools to empower individuals to lead lives of health freedom and resilience.

In essence, the integration of advanced laboratory services, high-tech healthcare tools, and digital resources into the fabric of healthcare delivery heralds a new era of health empowerment and autonomy. By equipping individuals with the means to leverage technology for self-education, self-diagnosis, and self-care, governments lay the groundwork for a healthcare revolution where every individual can access the tools and information needed to make informed healthcare decisions. This paradigm shift towards personalized, data-driven healthcare models ensures that no one is left behind due to financial constraints or lack of access to quality medical services, underscoring the imperative for governments to champion technological innovation to safeguard public health and well-being.

The transformative potential of advancing laboratory services and healthcare technologies to empower individuals to become their own health advocates underscores the ethos of health democratization and accessibility. By democratizing access to cutting-edge healthcare tools, governments foster a culture of health literacy, proactive health management, and preventive care, enabling individuals to take ownership of their well-being and thrive in a world where health freedom is a universal right. This vision of a society where individuals are empowered to navigate their health journeys with confidence, knowledge, and agency underscores the transformative power of technology in reshaping healthcare systems and ensuring equitable access to quality medical services for all.

Chapter Thirteen: Vital Insights: The Whispering Truth within Our Veins Revealed through Blood Chemistry

As our bodies whisper signs of discomfort and unease, it is our responsibility to listen. When unusual sensations or pains flutter within us, it is often easy to dismiss them, attributing them to fleeting causes or stress. Yet, in the intricate dance of our physiology, these whispers can reveal profound truths about our health. In these moments of uncertainty, we hold the key to unlocking vital insights through a simple yet profound action: a blood chemistry test.

The corridors of health centers, hospitals, and clinics stand as beacons of knowledge and security, offering a sanctuary for those seeking answers within the depths of their veins. The act of offering up a fraction of oneself to the laboratory gods is a ritual that bridges the gap between the unknown and the discernible. It is here, in the hallowed halls of diagnostics, that the canvas of our health is painted with precision and clarity.

Upon receiving the precious vial of crimson life, the journey of revelation begins. The blood, a fluid storyteller of our inner workings, holds within it the secrets of our well-being. As the meticulous analysis unfolds, a tapestry of numbers and markers emerges, each one a clue in the grand puzzle of our existence. Through the lens of science and technology, the veil is lifted, exposing the truths that lie beneath the surface.

With the results in hand, a sacred pact is forged between individual and knowledge. Armed with the intricate details of their inner landscape, individuals are empowered to chart a course towards optimal health. From cholesterol levels to glucose markers, each piece of data serves as a beacon guiding the way towards informed choices and tailored interventions.

In the realm of health, knowledge is power, and in the realm of blood chemistry tests, knowledge is enlightenment. The revelations gleaned from these tests are not merely numbers on a page; they are the whispers of our bodies translated into a language we can comprehend. Armed with this newfound wisdom, individuals possess the tools to sculpt their health destiny with precision and purpose.

As the veil of ignorance is lifted, a newfound sense of agency and empowerment blooms within. No longer are health outcomes dictated by chance or fate; they are sculpted by the choices we make armed with knowledge. The journey towards optimal health is no longer a nebulous dream but a tangible reality within reach, waiting to be grasped by those who dare to seek it.

In the tapestry of health, the threads of prevention are woven with the strands of awareness. Through the lens of a blood chemistry test, individuals are granted a glimpse into the future, a harbinger of potential pitfalls and opportunities for growth. Armed with this foresight, they march forward with clarity and purpose, intent on shaping a healthier tomorrow.

The journey towards health is not a solitary one but a communal endeavor, shared between individual and practitioner. In the halls of healthcare facilities, a symphony of collaboration unfolds, with healthcare providers and patients joining hands in the pursuit of well-being. Through the lens of shared knowledge and mutual understanding, the journey towards optimal health becomes a collective triumph.

In the crucible of self-discovery, the flames of resilience are kindled. Armed with the revelations unearthed through a blood chemistry test, individuals embark on a journey of transformation and renewal. With each choice made in alignment with their newfound insights, they take a step closer towards the pinnacle of health and vitality.

In the 13th chapter of my book, the importance of individuals seeking a blood chemistry test at a reputable healthcare center, hospital, or clinic is emphasized. The narrative delves into the significance of promptly addressing any unusual discomfort or pain experienced by the body through this essential medical examination. It portrays the ease with which one can access this service simply by choosing a trusted facility where they can generously provide a blood sample for detailed laboratory analysis.

As the story unfolds, readers are led through the process of obtaining their blood chemistry results and the critical role this information plays in understanding the inner workings of their bodies. The chapter vividly describes how individuals take the time to meticulously study these results, absorbing the intricate details that unveil the true state of their health. By gaining insights into their blood chemistry, they are equipped with valuable knowledge that empowers them to develop sophisticated strategies aimed at optimizing their well-being.

The narrative underscores the transformative impact of this proactive approach to healthcare, illustrating how individuals can leverage the information gleaned from their blood chemistry test to make informed decisions about their health. Armed with a comprehensive understanding of their body's dynamics, they embark on a journey towards optimal wellness, determined to navigate any health challenges with resilience and clarity. The overarching message resonates with the idea that by taking charge of their health through regular blood chemistry assessments, individuals can steer their well-being towards a trajectory of complete vitality.

Throughout the chapter, the narrative paints a compelling picture of individuals embracing the opportunity to proactively manage their health by prioritizing regular blood chemistry testing. It advocates for a paradigm shift towards a health-conscious mindset, urging readers to recognize the inherent value in monitoring their body's biochemical markers as a proactive measure towards wellness. The narrative eloquently portrays the empowerment that comes with knowledge, emphasizing how the insights derived from a blood chemistry test serve as a guiding light in crafting personalized health strategies.

In a world where health is often taken for granted, the chapter serves as a poignant reminder of the transformative potential embedded in a simple yet profound act of undergoing a blood chemistry test. It underscores the domino effect that arises from prioritizing one's health, rippling outwards to positively impact various facets of one's life. The narrative weaves together themes of empowerment, knowledge, and resilience, painting a vivid portrait of individuals who seize the opportunity to embrace their health journey with vigor and determination.

As the chapter unfolds, it invites readers to reflect on their own attitudes towards health and wellness, nudging them towards a mindset shift that prioritizes proactive healthcare measures. The narrative serves as a catalyst for introspection, prompting individuals to consider how they can leverage the insights from a blood chemistry test to tailor their lifestyle choices towards optimal health. Through evocative storytelling and compelling imagery, the chapter conveys a powerful message of self-care and empowerment, setting the stage for a transformative journey towards holistic well-being.

From the initial decision to undergo a blood chemistry test to the profound implications of understanding one's health status, the chapter navigates through a narrative tapestry that underscores the profound impact of proactive health management. It elucidates the notion that by embracing the opportunity to decode their body's intricate signals through a blood chemistry test, individuals are better equipped to embark on a journey of self-discovery and holistic healing. The chapter culminates in a crescendo of empowerment and self-realization, highlighting the immense potential that lies within each individual to steer their health towards a path of vitality and well-being.

In the 13th chapter of my book, it's crucial to emphasize the importance of individuals proactively seeking a blood chemistry test when they experience any unusual discomfort or pain in their body. Encouraging people to visit a well-standardized health care center, hospital, or clinic for this essential test serves as a pivotal step towards maintaining optimal health and wellbeing. By highlighting the convenience of these facilities in offering laboratory blood chemistry tests, readers can be motivated to take charge of their health with ease.

Moreover, the significance of receiving accurate and detailed blood chemistry results cannot be understated. When individuals actively engage in understanding the intricacies of their test results, they gain valuable insight into the inner workings of their bodies. This knowledge empowers them to craft highly effective strategies aimed at addressing any health concerns or imbalances that may be identified through the test results. By taking the time to analyze the data provided by the blood chemistry test, individuals pave the way for comprehensive and targeted health interventions.

Additionally, stressing the importance of interpreting blood chemistry results in a thorough and informed manner can guide individuals towards making informed decisions about their health. Equipped with a comprehensive understanding of their body's chemistry, individuals can tailor their lifestyle choices, dietary habits, and medical interventions to promote optimal health outcomes. This proactive approach to health management ensures that individuals are actively involved in shaping their health journey towards a state of complete wellness.

Furthermore, by highlighting the transformative potential of blood chemistry testing, individuals can be inspired to prioritize their health and well-being. Recognizing that a simple blood test can provide profound insights into one's health status encourages individuals to overcome any hesitations or concerns they may have about undergoing testing. This proactive stance towards health empowers individuals to take control of their well-being and make informed decisions that positively impact their overall health and vitality.

Moreover, underscoring the seamless process of obtaining a blood chemistry test at reputable healthcare facilities underscores the accessibility of this essential health evaluation. By emphasizing that individuals can easily access this service at established healthcare centers, hospitals, or clinics, readers are encouraged to prioritize their health without facing unnecessary barriers or challenges. This streamlined approach to obtaining a blood chemistry test emphasizes the simplicity and effectiveness of taking proactive steps towards better health.

Additionally, highlighting the value of regular blood chemistry testing as a preventive measure against potential health issues can instill a sense of responsibility towards health maintenance.

By incorporating routine blood tests into one's healthcare regimen, individuals can catch potential health concerns early and take proactive steps to address them. This preventive approach to health management underscores the proactive nature of individuals in safeguarding their well-being and longevity.

Furthermore, underscoring the role of blood chemistry testing in facilitating early detection of underlying health issues underscores the importance of proactive health monitoring. Encouraging individuals to undergo regular blood tests empowers them to detect and address potential health concerns before they escalate into more serious conditions. This proactive stance towards health maintenance highlights the invaluable benefits of preventive health measures in promoting long-term wellness and vitality.

Moreover, emphasizing the transformative impact of understanding one's blood chemistry results on overall health outcomes underscores the significance of informed decision-making in health management. By encouraging individuals to delve into the details of their test results and seek professional guidance where necessary, they can develop personalized strategies for optimizing their health. This attentive and proactive approach to health management enables individuals to make empowered choices that support their well-being and longevity.

Additionally, driving home the message that proactive engagement with blood chemistry testing can lead to significant improvements in one's health status underscores the profound impact of informed health decisions. By advocating for a proactive approach to health management through regular blood tests, individuals are empowered to take charge of their well-being and make informed decisions that positively impact their health outcomes. This proactive stance towards health underscores the transformative potential of proactive health monitoring in achieving optimal health and vitality.

The 13th chapter of my book serves as a vital reminder of the importance of individuals undergoing blood chemistry testing when experiencing any unusual symptoms. By encouraging individuals to seek out reputable healthcare facilities for these tests and actively engage with their results, my narrative effectively motivates readers to prioritize their health and well-being. Through a combination of informed decision-making, proactive health monitoring, and preventive measures, individuals are inspired to take control of their health journey and work towards achieving a state of optimal wellness.

In the concluding chapter of my book, it's imperative to emphasize the importance of regular blood chemistry tests as a vital component of proactive healthcare. Encouraging readers to visit reputable healthcare facilities, hospitals, or clinics for such tests can significantly contribute to early detection and prevention of health issues. By advocating for individuals to prioritize their health by obtaining these tests upon experiencing any unusual symptoms, you are inherently fostering a culture of self-care and preventative measures.

By facilitating easy access to blood chemistry tests, individuals can obtain valuable insights into their overall health status. The prompt availability of test results enables them to gain a deeper understanding of their body's inner workings, empowering them to make well-informed decisions regarding their health. This knowledge serves as a foundation for developing personalized strategies to address any health concerns effectively.

Through the act of obtaining and analyzing blood chemistry test results, individuals are equipped with the information necessary to tailor their lifestyle choices and healthcare decisions accordingly. Armed with a comprehensive understanding of their body's biochemical composition, readers are better positioned to make proactive choices that promote optimal health and well-being. This proactive approach can lead to the formulation of targeted, high-quality health strategies capable of driving significant improvements in their overall health.

The holistic understanding gained from blood chemistry tests helps individuals to identify potential health risks at an early stage, enabling them to implement preventive measures promptly. This proactive stance towards health management empowers individuals to take control of their well-being, reducing the likelihood of developing serious health conditions. Armed with the knowledge obtained from these tests, readers can make informed decisions that support their journey towards achieving optimal health outcomes.

By underscoring the significance of regular blood chemistry tests, you are advocating for a proactive stance towards health maintenance that is both empowering and enlightening. Encouraging readers to leverage the accessibility of healthcare facilities for their blood tests fosters a culture of wellness and personal responsibility. This initiative lays the groundwork for individuals to take charge of their health outcomes by proactively monitoring their biochemical parameters and responding appropriately to any anomalies detected.

Promoting the idea of studying blood chemistry results as a critical step in the journey towards improved health underscores the value of self-awareness and health literacy. By delving into the intricacies of their test results, individuals can decipher vital information about their health status and take necessary actions to optimize their well-being. This commitment to self-inquiry and understanding sets the stage for a holistic approach to health management that emphasizes prevention and informed decision-making.

The act of engaging with blood chemistry results not only provides individuals with valuable insights into their current health status but also serves as a catalyst for transformative change. Armed with a comprehensive understanding of their biochemical profile, readers can craft personalized health strategies that are tailored to their unique needs and circumstances. This proactive approach enables individuals to address underlying health issues effectively and embark on a journey towards sustainable wellness.

Encouraging readers to take the time to interpret their blood chemistry results reinforces the notion that health is a personal journey that requires active participation and commitment. By investing in the process of understanding their test results, individuals demonstrate a dedication to their well-being and a willingness to make informed choices that support their health goals. This deliberate engagement with their health data positions individuals as active agents in their healthcare journey, capable of driving positive change and realizing significant health improvements.

In conclusion, the emphasis on the significance of blood chemistry tests as a means of gaining valuable insights into one's health status underscores the transformative potential of proactive healthcare practices. By encouraging readers to proactively seek out these tests and engage with their results, you are fostering a culture of health literacy and self-empowerment. Through this proactive engagement with their health data, individuals can pave the way for improved health outcomes, enabling them to lead healthier, more fulfilling lives.

Chapter Fourteen: Empowering Health Freedom: Government-Driven Healthcare Security in Surgical, Dental, and Cancer Services

As the world navigates the complexities of the modern healthcare landscape, the for governments to meticulously engineer robust and comprehensive security systems to safeguard the pursuit of uncompromised health freedom emerges as an unequivocal necessity. Within this crucible of healthcare governance, the 14th chapter embarks upon a profound exploration of the intrinsic link between unassailable healthcare security and the fundamental rights of individuals to access surgical, dental, and cancer services safely and without reservation. This chapter serves as a powerful treatise delineating the pivotal role of governmental commitment in fortifying the sanctity of these crucial healthcare domains, underlining the indelible importance of engendering a climate where individuals can seek these vital services assured of their safety and well-being.

Amid the labyrinthine tapestry of healthcare provisions, the 14th chapter unfurls a compelling narrative, contoured by the imperative for governments to orchestrate stringent security measures tethered to surgical, dental, and cancer healthcare services. This narrative amplifies the urgency for governments to fortify the very bedrock of these healthcare realms, cultivating an environment where individuals can confidently seek these services, cognizant of the protective shield woven by resolute security frameworks. The chapter addresses the palpable impact of impregnable healthcare security, elucidating how it intersects with the ethos of health freedom, thereby fortifying the edifice of healthcare rights and individual autonomy.

As the 14th chapter unspools its eloquent exposition, it meticulously navigates the labyrinthine interplay between healthcare security and the unassailable right of individuals to access surgery, dentistry, and cancer services without trepidation or compromise. This scholarly discourse converges upon the indispensable role of government in erecting impregnable healthcare security architectures, bolstering the foundations upon which individuals can confidently partake in these pivotal healthcare domains. The chapter underscores the convergence of individual health freedom and the robust security apparatus meticulously engineered by governments, establishing a symbiotic relationship between these entities that underpins the fabric of a progressive healthcare ecosystem.

The 14th chapter cogently articulates the ethical imperative for governments to zealously institute fail-safe security measures surrounding surgery, dentistry, and cancer healthcare services, thereby reinforcing the cardinal principle of health freedom. This contemplative discourse expounds upon the symbiotic relationship between unfettered access to these critical healthcare domains and the unyielding assurance of security and well-being. By accentuating the pivotal role of governments in fortifying the sanctity of these healthcare realms, the chapter elucidates the transformative potential embedded within the fusion of health freedom with impenetrable security measures, fostering an environment where healthcare rights are inviolably upheld.

In the 14th chapter of this groundbreaking text, a deep dive into the critical importance of government intervention in fortifying the healthcare infrastructure unfolds. The narrative meticulously unravels the intricate web of complexities surrounding the imperative need for governments to labor ceaselessly towards establishing a world-class security framework. This chapter serves as a clarion call for heightened vigilance in safeguarding the sanctity of healthcare services, particularly in the domains of surgery, dentistry, and cancer treatment, where individuals place their most vital trusts.

The chapter elucidates how the very essence of health freedom hangs in delicate equilibrium, contingent upon the robust security measures enacted by governments across the globe. The text paints a vivid portrait of the vulnerabilities inherent in healthcare systems, underscoring the profound impact of breaches in security on individual well-being and public health at large. It delves into the myriad risks and challenges that accompany the delivery of critical healthcare services, emphasizing the indispensable role of governmental oversight in ensuring the unfettered access to safe, effective, and trustworthy healthcare provisions.

Furthermore, the narrative delves into the multifaceted spectrum of threats that loom ominously over the landscape of healthcare security. From cyber threats to physical vulnerabilities, the chapter navigates through the labyrinthine intricacies of safeguarding sensitive healthcare data, protecting physical healthcare facilities, and fortifying the integrity of treatment protocols. It underscores the imperative need for governments to adopt a proactive stance in preempting potential risks and fortifying the defenses of healthcare systems against evolving threats.

Moreover, the chapter unveils the ripple effects of lapses in healthcare security, shedding light on the far-reaching consequences of compromised healthcare services. It delves into the profound disruptions that ensue when individuals are deprived of access to safe and reliable healthcare provisions, accentuating the cascading impact on individual health outcomes and societal well-being. This exploration serves as a poignant reminder of the paramount significance of robust security measures in safeguarding the fundamental rights of individuals to quality healthcare services.

The text meticulously details the intricate dance between governmental authorities and healthcare stakeholders in coalescing efforts towards bolstering healthcare security. It elucidates the synergistic partnerships required to fortify the defense mechanisms of healthcare systems, advocating for collaborative endeavors aimed at mitigating risks and enhancing resilience. The narrative underscores the pivotal role of coordinated action in fortifying the healthcare ecosystem and safeguarding the sanctity of healthcare services for all individuals.

The chapter weaves a tapestry of urgency and gravity, painting a vivid picture of the stakes at hand in the realm of healthcare security. It underscores the critical need for governments to redouble their efforts in elevating healthcare security to unparalleled levels of excellence, ensuring that individuals can access surgical, dental, and cancer healthcare services with unwavering confidence. The narrative serves as a compelling call to action, urging governments to allocate resources, enact stringent regulations, and foster collaboration to fortify the bulwarks of healthcare security and uphold the fundamental tenets of health freedom.

The 14th chapter of this enlightening text serves as a poignant testament to the indelible importance of robust healthcare security systems in upholding the sacred trust between individuals and healthcare providers. It delves into the profound implications of lapses in security, articulating the far-reaching consequences of compromised healthcare services on individual health outcomes and public health. Through a meticulous examination of the challenges and imperatives of healthcare security, the chapter imparts a powerful message on the indispensable role of governments in ensuring the integrity, reliability, and accessibility of healthcare services in the domains of surgery, dentistry, and cancer treatment.

Chapter 14 delves into the critical importance of robust security systems in healthcare settings, focusing particularly on the domains of surgery, dentistry, and cancer treatments. Governments play a pivotal role in ensuring the safety and security of individuals seeking these essential healthcare services, as the integrity of these procedures directly impacts individuals' well-being. Therefore, the chapter emphasizes the urgent need for governments to prioritize the establishment of top-tier security mechanisms to guarantee unparalleled health freedom for all individuals accessing such services.

At the forefront of the discussion is the inherent vulnerability individuals face when undergoing surgical procedures, dental treatments, or cancer therapies. Given the invasive nature of these interventions and the potential risks involved, it is imperative for governments to implement stringent security measures to safeguard patients' health and prevent any untoward incidents or malpractices. By creating a high-caliber security framework, governments can instill confidence in individuals seeking these critical healthcare services, assuring them of their safety and well-being throughout their medical journeys.

The chapter underscores how the efficacy of surgery, dentistry, and cancer treatments hinges significantly on the establishment of secure healthcare environments. By fortifying security protocols within hospitals, clinics, and specialized healthcare centers, governments can mitigate risks, deter potential threats, and enhance the overall quality of care provided to patients. This comprehensive approach not only ensures the physical safety of individuals but also cultivates an environment conducive to optimal health outcomes and patient recovery.

The chapter further highlights the ethical imperative of upholding stringent security standards in healthcare settings, particularly in the context of surgery, dentistry, and cancer treatments. Ensuring the confidentiality of patient information, maintaining the integrity of medical procedures, and safeguarding individuals against any form of malpractice or negligence are paramount responsibilities that governments must uphold. By establishing a robust security infrastructure, governments demonstrate their commitment to ethical healthcare practices and prioritize the well-being of their citizens above all else.

The chapter explores the multifaceted benefits of investing in high-quality security systems for surgery, dentistry, and cancer healthcare services. Not only do stringent security measures protect patients from potential harm or exploitation, but they also bolster the reputation of healthcare facilities and inspire trust in the healthcare system as a whole. By cultivating a culture of safety and security, governments can foster a conducive environment for medical practitioners to deliver superior care and for individuals to access healthcare services with confidence and peace of mind.

Additionally, the chapter delves into the intricate interplay between regulatory frameworks and security protocols in healthcare settings. Governments are tasked with enacting and enforcing regulations that dictate the standards of care, safety, and security within healthcare facilities offering surgery, dentistry, and cancer treatments. By harmonizing regulatory requirements with robust security measures, governments can uphold the highest standards of healthcare quality, protect patient rights, and minimize the risks associated with medical procedures in these specialized fields.

An essential aspect highlighted in the chapter is the role of technology in augmenting security systems within healthcare environments. Advancements in digital security, biometric authentication, surveillance technologies, and access control systems offer unprecedented opportunities for governments to enhance the security of surgery, dentistry, and cancer healthcare services. By leveraging cutting-edge technologies, governments can fortify security measures, streamline healthcare operations, and elevate the standard of care provided to individuals seeking these critical medical treatments.

The chapter underscores the significance of international collaboration and knowledge exchange in strengthening security systems for surgery, dentistry, and cancer healthcare services. Given the global nature of healthcare challenges and the universal need for robust security protocols, governments can benefit greatly from sharing best practices, expertise, and resources with international partners. By engaging in collaborative initiatives, governments can enrich their security frameworks, innovate new strategies, and collectively work towards ensuring universal access to safe and high-quality healthcare services for all individuals.

The chapter addresses the imperative of transparency and accountability in healthcare security systems, emphasizing the importance of regular audits, compliance checks, and monitoring mechanisms to uphold the integrity of security protocols. By fostering a culture of transparency and accountability, governments can demonstrate their commitment to ensuring the safety and well-being of individuals accessing surgery, dentistry, and cancer healthcare services. This ethos of openness and accountability not only engenders trust in the healthcare system but also promotes a culture of continual improvement and excellence in healthcare delivery.

Chapter 14 serves as a call to action for governments worldwide to prioritize the establishment of top-tier security systems to ensure a hundred percent health freedom for individuals seeking surgery, dentistry, and cancer healthcare services. By investing in robust security measures, enacting stringent regulatory frameworks, leveraging cutting-edge technologies, fostering international collaboration, and promoting transparency and accountability, governments can create a secure and conducive environment for individuals to access essential healthcare services with confidence, safety, and peace of mind. This concerted effort to fortify healthcare security not only protects individuals from harm and exploitation but also underscores governments' unwavering commitment to upholding the highest standards of ethical healthcare practices and safeguarding the well-being of their citizens.

As individuals navigate the intricate landscape of healthcare choices, the pivotal role of governments in fostering a robust security infrastructure becomes glaringly evident. The intersection of surgery, dentistry, and cancer health services marks crucial junctures where people place implicit trust in the healthcare system. Governments, therefore, bear the onus of constructing unparalleled security measures to safeguard the sanctity of these essential services, ensuring that individuals can access them with unwavering confidence.

Against the backdrop of escalating healthcare complexities, the demand for stringent security protocols within surgery, dentistry, and cancer healthcare is paramount. By instituting comprehensive strategies that encompass technological advancements, regulatory frameworks, and oversight mechanisms, governments can fortify the foundations of healthcare delivery. This proactive stance not only inspires trust but also reinforces the imperative of health freedom as a fundamental human right.

The convergence of surgical interventions, dental procedures, and cancer treatments underscores the criticality of upholding the highest standards of security within healthcare systems. Governments must steer their efforts toward orchestrating multi-faceted security measures that encompass data protection, patient privacy, facility regulations, and personnel training. Such an integrated approach not only bolsters the resilience of healthcare infrastructures but also underscores the unwavering commitment to ensuring the safety and well-being of individuals seeking vital healthcare services.

In the realm of surgery, dentistry, and cancer healthcare, the imperatives of safety, efficacy, and patient-centric care converge to form the bedrock of healthcare quality. Governments must champion the cause of health freedom by enshrining stringent security measures that uphold the sanctity of these services. Through meticulous planning, collaboration with healthcare stakeholders, and continuous evaluation, governments can forge a healthcare ecosystem where individuals can access transformative healthcare services with unparalleled peace of mind.

The complexity inherent in surgical procedures, dental treatments, and cancer care necessitates a meticulous approach to security implementation within healthcare systems. Governments must proactively engage in crafting and enforcing regulations that mirror international best practices, integrating cutting-edge technologies and expertise to create resilient security frameworks. This concerted effort not only bolsters the integrity of healthcare services but also fortifies the foundation of health freedom as a cornerstone of modern healthcare governance.

At the heart of effective healthcare governance lies the commitment to upholding the primacy of patient safety and empowerment. Governments must be unwavering in their resolve to institute stringent security measures that safeguard individuals accessing surgical, dental, and cancer healthcare services. By fostering a culture of accountability, transparency, and collaboration within healthcare systems, governments lay the groundwork for a healthcare landscape where individuals can exercise their health autonomy without compromise.

The synergy between governmental initiatives and healthcare security underscores the symbiotic relationship between public policy and healthcare delivery. In elevating the security standards within surgery, dentistry, and cancer healthcare, governments pave the way for a healthcare environment predicated on trust, accountability, and patient-centered care. This concerted effort not only redoubles the commitment to health freedom but also sets a precedent for robust healthcare governance that resonates across borders and disciplines.

The intricate interplay between healthcare security and governance underscores the indispensable role of governments in shaping the healthcare landscape. By devising comprehensive security mechanisms that mitigate risks, protect patient rights, and enhance healthcare quality, governments foster an environment where individuals can seek surgery, dentistry, and cancer services with unwavering confidence. This dedication to excellence not only amplifies the principles of health freedom but also underscores the government's profound commitment to prioritizing public health and well-being.

As healthcare systems evolve to meet the demands of a dynamic healthcare landscape, the imperative of government-led security measures within surgery, dentistry, and cancer services assumes paramount significance. Governments must proactively champion the cause of health freedom by spearheading initiatives that secure the integrity of these essential healthcare domains. Through relentless dedication to advancing healthcare security, governments lay the foundation for a healthcare ecosystem where individuals can access life-transforming healthcare services with unparalleled security and peace of mind.

In conclusion, the profound impact of robust security measures within surgery, dentistry, and cancer healthcare reverberates far beyond clinical settings. Governments play a pivotal role in shaping the contours of healthcare governance, underscoring the significance of upholding rigorous security standards that safeguard patient interests, enhance healthcare quality, and uphold the principles of health freedom. By steadfastly championing the cause of healthcare security, governments not only fortify the pillars of healthcare governance but also reaffirm their commitment to ensuring that individuals can access essential healthcare services with unwavering trust and confidence.

www.ingramcontent.com/pod-product-compliance
Lightning Source LLC
Chambersburg PA
CBHW050315230526
45471CB00005B/2197